Beta-Carotene

Beta-Carotene

How it Can Help You to Better Health

Caroline Wheater

Thorsons
An Imprint of HarperCollins*Publishers*

Thorsons
An Imprint of GraftonBooks
A Division of HarperCollins*Publishers*
77-85 Fulham Palace Road,
Hammersmith, London W6 8JB

Published by Thorsons 1991
10 9 8 7 6 5 4 3 2 1

A CIP catalogue record for this book
is available from the British Library

ISBN 0 7225 2445 5

Typeset by Harper Phototypesetters Limited,
Northampton, England
Printed in Great Britain by
HarperCollinsManufacturing, Glasgow

Contents

Acknowledgements

I would like to extend my thanks to those health professionals who gave me valuable time, advice and information while writing this book. Without their dedication beta-carotene would still be off the map.

Ursula Arens, Professor Ami Ben-Amotz, Dr Adrianne Bendich, Dr Gladys Block, Dr Graham Burton, Dr David Forman, Professor Charles Hennekens, Professor Norman Krinsky, Professor John Marks, Professor Micheline Mathews-Roth, Maxwell Noble, Dr Richard Peto, Dr Tom Sanders, Professor Leonida Santamaria, Professor Hans Stich, Dr David Thurnham, Amanda Ursell, Professor John Weisburger and Dr Regina Ziegler.

I would like to voice special gratitude for invaluable scientific guidance to Dr George Brittan, Professor Anthony Diplock and Dr Catherine Rice-Evans.

Last but not least, thanks must go to Mum and Dad for their continuing love and support, and to my friends, who make it all worthwhile.

Foreword

The world in which we live is characterized by bright colours that give interest to our environment and increase our aesthetic enjoyment of our surroundings. From the brilliant colour of the homely tomato to the vivid colours of the Mexican quetzal, the carotenoid pigments provide a huge range of colours of great variety that are often responsible for controlling or determining animal behaviour, and that serve a vital purpose in protecting plants from the harmful effects of the sun's radiation. More than 600 carotenoid pigments have been identified, of which beta carotene is by far the most important. Carotenoids are also widely used in the food industry as very safe food colourants, and many everyday items in our diet have their appearance enhanced by the addition of beta carotene or other carotenoid pigments. Such pigments are also frequently used by the pharmaceutical industry to colour tablets.

Until quite recently the significance of beta carotene in human and animal health has been limited to an understanding of the fact that beta carotene and, to a lesser extent, other carotenoids serve as a nutritional precursor of vitamin A.

During the past decade there has been intensive research on the possible protective effect of certain nutrients against cardio-vascular disease and certain forms of cancer. A major factor in the natural history of these diseases is the formation of certain molecules (that are chemically highly reactive) which interfere with normal cellular chemistry to cause changes which manifest themselves as disease. These reactive chemicals, called free radicals, are usually generated from active forms of the oxygen in the air we breathe, themselves free radicals which are formed as random events alongside normal, life-giving, cellular respiration.

The control by 'antioxidant nutrients' of these randomly generated free radicals has become an absorbing interest to biochemists and medical scientists. The classic 'antioxidant nutrients' are vitamins A, C and E and the minerals selenium, manganese, copper and zinc which are required in minute quantities in the human diet.

Recent research has indicated that beta carotene, and other carotenoids, also contribute to the sophisticated and complex protective mechanism that prevents free radical damage. In the test tube under laboratory conditions it can readily be demonstrated that carotenoids may trap and neutralize active forms of oxygen, but this is a long way from showing that carotenoids have any significance in human health, apart from their vitamin A precursor role, in contributing to the defence of the body against oxidants. However, exciting research is now being reported which indicates that those persons who have a large amount of fresh fruits and vegetables in their diet, and in whom the body level of carotenoids is high, are significantly less likely to suffer from cardiovascular disease and certain forms of cancer in later life. The prevention of disease by nutritional means is thus a significant consideration that may prove to have profound consequences for public health.

In Caroline Wheater's comprehensive review of current knowledge on beta carotene, she gives details about the sources and chemistry of beta carotene, the nutritional significance of the compound, and of its potential role as a chemopreventive agent in the natural history of cancer and cardiovascular disease. Her book is essentialy for the general reader, but it also provides excellent background reading for the scientist interested in this fascinating subject for whom a selection of original references for further reading is also given.

PROFESSOR ANTHONY I. DIPLOCK PH.D., D.SC.
Chairman, Division of Biochemistry
University of London, Guy's Hospital, London

Introduction

What is Beta-Carotene?

Most colours in nature are derived from pigments, from the tiniest ladybird's shell to the largest Redwood tree. Pigments make life visually interesting. They create contrasts – green leaves against brown soil, or a climbing pink rose against a white wall – and they also provide camouflage – a sandy lion hunting in the dry grasslands of Africa, or a chameleon merging into violet blossom. Life would be very dull indeed if all we could see were shades of grey.

We rarely stop to think about it, but pigments add a unique dimension to our lives. Both synthetic and natural, they are everywhere: in the fruitbowl; in the greenhouse; printed in books, money and furnishings; painted on cars; even dictating the looks of the family pet! Stone Age humans expressed themselves by drawing paintings on cave walls using vivid colours derived from plants and rocks. Different colours suit different moods, and are a vital influence over our perception of the world.

Plant Pigments

Beta-carotene makes an enormous contribution to the colours we see around us. It is a pigment manufactured in plants, algae and bacteria, and it gives colour to many of the foods we eat, including carrots, apricots and oranges, to name but a few.

In its pure, crystallized form, it is red or purple – depending on the source – but is often the main pigment in orange coloured fruits and vegetables. Beta-carotene is also present in dark green leafy vegetables, but cannot be seen because it is hidden by the green chlorophyll (the substance which creates energy for the plant).

Beta-carotene is just one pigment in a huge colour palette seen throughout nature. It is part of a large and important family of pigments called the carotenoids; these pigments are widely distributed in the plant kingdom and can determine the colour of animals that feed on them too. Every year plants produce an estimated 100 million tonnes of carotenoids.

So far, scientists have identified 600 different carotenoids, which together make up a rainbow of colours and are responsible for the often brilliant yellows and reds seen in flowers and fruit. The highest concentration of any carotenoid is found in the pheasant's eye narcissus flower, where beta-carotene can constitute up to 16 per cent of the dry weight. The daily rate of beta-carotene formation in this narcissus is over 10,000 times that in carrots.[1]

However, carotenoids do not exist simply to make the world look colourful. They serve an integral purpose in keeping a plant healthy, and do this in two ways. First, beta-carotene protects the plant from burning up under the sun's rays. When humans go out in the sun, a substance called melanin is produced in the epidermis to protect the skin, and this causes suntans. As humans produce melanin, so plants produce beta-carotene; its job is to mop up the excess energy which has been absorbed by chlorophyll, but which the plant does not need. Without such a mopping up substance, excess energy can create a highly reactive molecule called singlet oxygen (see Chapter 8) which can damage plant cells.

A good example of this first function of beta-carotene is in the alga *Dunaliella bardawil*. It has an extremely large capacity for manufacturing beta-carotene when it is in very salty, hot conditions. On dunaliella farms (in Australia, Israel and Hawaii) acres of bright orange algae are stretched out, soaking up the sun. The more the sun shines the more orange the algae turn, frantically producing beta-carotene to stop damage to their cells.

The other main function of carotenoids is light-harvesting. Lutein and fucoxanthin, for example, allow plants to pick up different wavelengths of light. Fucoxanthin is present in seaweeds allowing them to absorb extra light, since the sea can obscure light and make it difficult to trap enough to remain healthy.

The Study of Carotenoids

Scientists first became interested in the carotenoids during the nineteenth century. In 1831 a scientist named Wackenroder isolated beta-carotene, and in 1837 Berzelius pinpointed the yellow pigment of autumn leaves as the carotenoid lutein. Between 1900 and 1927, researchers headed by Tswett and Willstatter managed to work out procedures for the separation of carotene, lycopene, lutein, fucoxanthin and bixin.

It was also during this period that beta-carotene was established as being the main source of vitamin A for animals. Beta-carotene also makes up a large proportion of the human intake of vitamin A, especially for vegetarians. Approximately fifty other carotenoids can be converted by the body into vitamin A, but none as effectively as beta-carotene.

The study of carotenoids has seen a boom in the last forty years. In 1930, scientists knew of only 15 different varieties; modern techniques, such as high-performance liquid chromatography (HPLC), have made it possible to take that total to 600. HPLC can identify the number of compounds contained in one small test-tube with amazing accuracy, and display the results using computer graphics.

The formation of carotenoids seems to have begun very early in the history of the world; algae and bacteria were among the earliest forms of life, and are all capable of manufacturing essential carotenoids. In fact algae and bacteria contain a much wider and more complex group of carotenoids than the higher forms of plant life; and consequently we don't come across many of these carotenoids in our diet.

Out of the 600 identified carotenoids, there are five major varieties: fucoxanthin, lutein, beta-carotene, violaxanthin and neoxanthin. Fucoxanthin is the pigment of many marine algae and brown seaweeds – bladderwrack for example – and it is the most abundant member of the family.

By comparison, other well-known carotenoids such as lycopene (found predominantly in tomatoes) and capsanthin (the pigment which colours peppers and chillies) have a limited occurrence. Some carotenoids, such as phytofluene and neurosporene, only exist in order to manufacture more important ones.

Carotenoids in the Animal Kingdom

Carotenoids are the most widely-occurring pigments in the animal kingdom after the melanins. They can be seen in mammals, fish, crustaceans, birds and insects. Certain animals, such as flamingos and ladybirds, are dependent on carotenoids for their entire colour; but no evidence has yet been found to show that animals can manufacture their own carotenoids – they must take them in as food.

Carotenoids occur in a wide variety of birds, particularly in their plumage. If birds kept in zoos are lacking in dietary carotenoids their plumage begins to fade. Flamingos in captivity have to be supplemented with synthetic canthaxanthin in order to keep their colour vibrant.

Carotenoids are also widely found in crustaceans whose diets contain so much algae. Lobsters don't eat algae, but they do eat smaller animals that rely on algae for food and therefore have a regular intake. Fresh lobsters are blue in colour; this is because astaxanthin, the main carotenoid inside their shells, is bound onto a protein which gives it a bluish tinge. Starfish obtain their bluish/pink colour from a derivative of astaxanthin. When heated these carotenoids change their chemical structure; that is why boiled lobsters and crabs are a deep pink colour.

Carotenoids in our Diet

In the human diet, it is possible to find up to one hundred different carotenoids, some in minute quantities. Estimates differ on how many types can be found in one person, and range from 20 to 40.[2] There are five main types which we eat regularly: beta-carotene, lutein, lycopene, cryptoxanthin and alpha-carotene. Some that appear in the diet less frequently are: zeaxanthin, capsanthin and astaxanthin. Every human population has different levels of each particular carotenoid, depending on which foods are staples.

In blood samples taken in the United Kingdom, proportions of beta-carotene and lutein are approximately equal, with lycopene coming a close third. Cryptoxanthin is the fourth most common, followed by alpha-carotene. In the United States the picture is different; there the tomato is the second most popular vegetable (after the potato) and because of this, blood levels of lycopene are likely to be the highest out of all carotenoids – up to 35 per cent. Lycopene is followed by beta-carotene and lutein – around 20 per cent each – and cryptoxanthin is next with 10 per cent.[3] In Hungary, blood samples are high in capsanthin because of the high levels of red peppers in the diet.

Beta-carotene is found in many orange and dark green leafy fruits and vegetables (see page 20). Lutein is often found in the same foods in similar amounts, but it is not found in carrots or red palm oil. Lycopene is the red pigment mainly found in tomatoes, which is also found in some fruits, including those of poisonous plants such as woody nightshade. As fruits ripen, a massive synthesis of carotenoids occurs: a stored tomato can produce 1.2 milligrams of lycopene a day.

Cryptoxanthin is found particularly in soft orange fruits such as apricots, peaches and papaya. Alpha-carotene is found in some green leafy vegetables, and in small amounts in carrots. Zeaxanthin is found in sweet corn and fruit; capsanthin in red peppers and chillies. Other more minor carotenoids can be found in all those vegetables too, but they are not so significant in terms of colour.

Once ingested, carotenoids are stored in several places in the body.[4] The main area for storage is the adipose (fatty) tissue, where between 80 and 85 per cent is stored. The liver contains between 8 and 12 per cent and the muscle just 2 to 3 per cent. The actual concentration of carotenoids is highest in the corpus luteum (a small organelle in the uterus, which releases hormones if an ovum is fertilized) and the adrenal gland.

Of the total 'body pool' of carotenoids, 1 per cent, on average, circulates in the blood. The levels depend on the quantity of pigment-containing foods, or supplements, ingested each day. Carotenoids are absorbed into the blood through the walls of the intestines and transported around the body by lipoproteins (which also transport lipids – fatty molecules – to the liver, and then on to fatty tissues).

Carotenoids as Additives

Natural extracts containing carotenoids have been used in cooking for centuries, including annatto (yellow), saffron (yellow), paprika (red), xanthophyll (yellow), carrot and red palm oil. In 1954 the first synthetic carotenoid was put onto the market as a food colouring. Beta-carotene was the chosen pigment, and the company responsible was Hoffmann-La Roche, which had spent many years researching carotenoids. Now, as well as providing beta-carotene for the food industry, Hoffman-La Roche also supplies pharmaceutical grades for use in dietary supplements and prescription medications.

Beta-carotene remains the main colourant for fat-based foods such as cheese, margarine and oils. It is safe, and used as a 'natural' alternative to the azo dyes (derived from coal-tar). In its natural state beta-carotene is fat soluble, i.e. it can only be dissolved by fat, but technologists have come up with ways to make it water soluble. This means that it can be used as a colourant in juices, drinks, dried soups, canned soups and gravies, yogurt, ice-cream, jellies, syrups, jams, sweets, pasta, egg products and meat products.

Beta-carotene and lutein are the two most commonly used carotenoids in animal feed; lutein gives a bright lemon-yellow colour, beta-carotene a more golden-yellow shade. They are used in cattle and poultry feed to affect the colour of skin, fat, egg yolk and beak. Astaxanthin is added to the feed of farmed salmon and trout, to give the fresh a natural pinky-orange colour.

Beta-carotene is often used in butter to even out the tones of colour. In the summer cows fed on pasture will be eating lots of lush grass, rich in beta-carotene, but in the winter they will eat cattle feed and their milk will lack that rich creamy colour. Beta-carotene has also been associated with fertility in cows: some studies have said that fertility is lowered if cows are denied access to fresh grass.

Canthaxanthin used to be fed to hens to improve the colour of yolks, but this practice is now being phased out due to concerns about its effects on human health. Tests have shown that canthaxanthin crystals can build up in the retina of the human eye, and that the crystals could be capable of breaking cells and damaging membranes. However, it is unlikely that canthaxanthin is harmful when taken in reasonable amounts; normal intake is less than 1 milligram (mg) a day, and the people who developed crystals were taking 200 mg every day for weeks.

Beta-Carotene, two of its derivatives, and canthaxanthin have several other, less common functions. They are used to colour sugar-coated tablets from yellow through deep orange, red-brown to red. They are also used in the colouration of cosmetic products, lotions, lipsticks and powder bases.

Specific Role in Health for Beta-Carotene

Apart from being widely used as a food additive, beta-carotene has several other important functions linked to human health. Its role as a safe form of vitamin A is primary. Humans and other mammals are able to convert beta-carotene into vitamin A. For some people a dietary intake of foods which contain beta-carotene is their only source of vitamin A, so fruits and vegetables rich in the nutrient are very valuable. Beta-carotene is unique amongst carotenoids in that it can form two molecules of vitamin A from each one of its own molecules.

However, whereas vitamin A can be toxic if taken in too large a quantity, an equivalent amount of beta-carotene is totally safe. Evidence for this has been collected over the past twenty years by treating the light-sensitivity condition known as erythro-poietic protoporphyria (EPP) with beta-carotene (see Chapter

4). People who have EPP have too many porphyrins – the light-sensitive pigments in the skin – which when exposed to light generate a volatile species of molecule called singlet oxygen. Singlet oxygen can cause damage to the cellular structure of skin and make it sore and red.

Massive doses of beta-carotene – up to 300 mg a day – for several years have not led to any bad side-effects, except for a slight yellowing of the skin, which most people like! Supplementing sufferers with beta-carotene results in an increased tolerance of sunlight. Just as beta-carotene protects plants from burning up, so it protects skin by quenching the free radicals produced by porphyrins. However, it cannot heal the condition totally.

Beta-carotene also has another built-in safeguard against toxicity; if your body has no need for extra vitamin A it will not be converted, it will simply be stored away in its digested state, or excreted. You can eat as many foods containing beta-carotene as you like, and you can take a beta-carotene supplement, with complete confidence that you won't overdose on vitamin A.

Following this dietary plan may do you more good than you realize; in addition to providing adequate amounts of vitamin A in the diet, beta-carotene is also under close scientific scrutiny by cancer experts. Beta-carotene is part of a new research thrust into finding *chemopreventive* nutrients. Chemoprevention means preventing cancer before it has even reared its ugly head. Chemopreventive nutrients are nutrients we eat in foods every day, and include vitamins C and E and minerals such as selenium.

Since the early 1980s, it has been suggested that beta-carotene is a key candidate for such a role. And not just because it can be converted into vitamin A. Scientists believe beta-carotene could be protective against cancer in its own right. Widespread scientific studies have linked low consumption of fruits and vegetables containing beta-carotene, and a low level of beta-carotene in the blood, to a higher risk of developing certain cancers, particularly lung cancer. The association is less significant, but still apparent, with cancers of the stomach and mouth. Initial experiments have also led scientists to believe that beta-carotene could have a beneficial effect on cancers of the skin, colon and bladder. (See Chapters 6 and 7.)

The reasons why beta-carotene could be protective are not yet clear, but much time and effort is going into researching the subject. Along with vitamins C and E, and the mineral selenium, beta-carotene is an antioxidant; this means that it can mop up free radicals. Free radicals are unbalanced molecules which can damage other molecules, and have been linked to all kinds of degenerative diseases such as cancer, rheumatoid arthritis and atherosclerosis.

Free radicals can initiate cancer by damaging DNA, and they can damage the vital enzymic processes which are essential to the workings of the body. It has also been demonstrated that beta-carotene can enhance the immune system (see Chapter 8 for a deeper discussion of the evidence). Beta-carotene is the most efficient quencher of singlet oxygen known; singlet oxygen is a very reactive state of the normally stable gas that we breathe. Because it has so much energy it can form free radicals as well as cause damage to cells.

Official health bodies all over the world are backing the concept that cancer is preventable in many cases. The National Cancer Institute in the United States, Europe Against Cancer and the German Society for Nutrition are all advising people to eat more fresh fruit and vegetables, particularly those containing beta-carotene. The influential American National Cancer Institute is funding research to look at the effects of beta-carotene on cancers of the lung, mouth, colon, skin and all other sites.

Scientists are also beginning to look at other carotenoids in the light of these new discoveries. Lutein, lycopene, crypto-xanthin and alpha-carotene are all being investigated for possible protective functions.

Beta-carotene is the success story of the carotenoid family, but the whole field is open to discovery, still as exciting and promising as it was over 150 years ago. Who would have guessed then that the identification of the solitary beta-carotene would lead to the discovery of 600 more relations present in hundreds of different living organisms? And who would have thought that something as humble as the pigment found in carrots could protect against lung cancer? Every tiny discovery has helped to put carotenoids on the road to recognition. This book looks at the stops along the way.

Notes

1. *Carotenoids*, Otto Isler (ed.), 1971, Birkhauser verlag, Basel and Stuttgart.
2. Parker, R.S., 'Carotenoid and tocopherol composition of human adipose tissue', *American Journal of Clinical Nutrition*, 1988, 47, pp. 33–6.
3. Lachance, P., 'Dietary intake of carotenes and the carotene gap', *Clinical Nutrition*, 1988, 7, 3, pp. 118–22.
4. Bendich, A. *et. al.*, 'Biological actions of carotenoids', *FASEB Journal*, 1989, 3, pp. 1927–32.

Chapter 1

The Sources of Beta-Carotene

Rich countries have rich diets; they also have very high rates of obesity, heart disease and cancer. This observation, increasingly seen in the years since the Second World War is beginning to change the foods we eat. People who once stuffed themselves on cream buns and trifle are gradually turning to healthier, lighter diets. Meat and dairy products – twenty years ago an essential part of everyday eating – are losing popularity, in favour of low fat, high fibre, fresh foods.

As change comes about, it is essential that non-animal sources of important vitamins and nutrients are eaten more regularly. Vitamin A is derived chiefly from liver and dairy products, it plays a vital role in keeping skin, cells and mucous membranes healthy. Beta-carotene is a safe and widely available source of vitamin A, it is found in fruits and vegetables, and this makes it ideal for vegans and lacto-vegetarians.

Fifty years ago the only way of consuming beta-carotene was through food. Nowadays it is available in supplement form too – go into any health food shop or chemist and you will see products such as VitaBrit and Healthcrafts beta-carotene gracing the selves.

Dietary Sources

Beta-carotene is in many types of fruit and vegetables, on the whole those containing it are either deep yellow/orange in colour or dark green and leafy. It can also be found in some animals, such as cows.

Yellow/orange vegetables	Dark green leafy vegetables	Yellow/orange fruits
Carrots	Spinach	Apricots
Sweet potatoes	Broccoli	Cantaloups
Pumpkins	Brussels sprouts	Papayas
Winter squash	Cabbage	Mangoes
	Kale	Carambolas
	Endive	Melons
	Chicory	Nectarines
	Escarole	Peaches
	Watercress	Oranges
	Green parts of beetroot	
	Turnip	
	Mustard	
	Dandelion	

Figure 1.1. Some examples of vegetables and fruit containing beta-carotene

The amount of beta-carotene found in food depends on the season, how ripe the food is and what type it is within its own particular family. Different types of the same vegetable family can have varying beta-carotene levels. Savoy cabbage contains 0.3 mg per 4 oz serving; spring cabbage has 0.5 mg per 4 oz serving – that's a 60 per cent difference. Iceberg lettuce has lower levels of beta-carotene than a traditional round lettuce; you will notice that the round lettuce has darker leaves – this is the beta-carotene.

Carrots

Carrots are a very important source of beta-carotene: in the United Kingdom they account for 60 per cent of intake. Compared to other commonly eaten vegetables they have the highest beta-carotene content. Within the carrot group, however, are large variations in levels. Some have almost twice as much as others. The colour of carrots increases during the growing season; young, small carrots, pale in colour, contain little beta-carotene. In the mature, ripe carrot, beta-carotene accounts for about 60 per cent of the total carotenoid content, alpha-carotene 20 per cent, and the rest is made up from lycopene and other relations of beta-carotene.

A study of carrots was carried out recently at the University of Helsinki. In Finland the carrot is one of the most important vegetables in the diet – the average daily intake is 18.3 grams per person. The carrot is a major part of Finnish agriculture, and good colour is essential for success at market. The deeper the colour the healthier the carrot because there is more beta-carotene available.[1]

The researcher running the study looked into the make-up of 19 different varieties of carrot and found that the varieties Nantes Notabene 370 and Nantes Fancy Notabene 405 were rich in both alpha- and beta-carotene. Narbonne, Nelson and Nantucket were high in beta-carotene, Berlicum R, a carrot used for cattle feed, was also high. The range of beta-carotene levels went from 4,600 microgramme (μg) per 100 g of fresh weight, to 10,300 μg.

Regardless of type the researcher found that all the carrots contained enough beta-carotene for a 100 g portion of fresh carrot to satisfy the recommended daily allowance of vitamin A. In Finland the carrot accounts for 10 per cent of the dietary intake of vitamin A.

The interest in beta-carotene as a possible protection against some cancers has prompted a number of studies to look into the carotenoid content of relevant vegetables and fruit. A recent analysis showed that fresh yellow and orange vegetables were very high in beta-carotene. In comparison fresh, green, leafy vegetables were moderately high in beta-carotene (10 to 20 per cent) but very high in lutein and related carotenoids (80 to 90 per cent).[2]

The study also found that lutein and relations are very susceptible to damage from cooking in a microwave, between 19 and 57 per cent of these carotenoids are destroyed when cooked in this way. On the other hand only 15 per cent of beta-carotene and related carotenoids are lost through microwaving.

During the study, the researchers confirmed that vegetables and fruits contained a mixture of carotenoids, although one tended to dominate. This led the researchers to conclude that 'Consumption of carotenoids in addition to beta-carotene may be associated with a lower risk of cancer.' The suggestion that other carotenoids may have a valuable role to play in cancer prevention is not new. The research has simply not yet been done.

Ranking	Fruit	Pounds per capita
1	Oranges	29.7
2	Bananas	22.2
3	Apples	20.8
4	Melons	20.2
5	Peaches	9.2
6	Grapefruit	8.2
7	Grapes	5.4
8	Pears	4.4
9	Strawberries	4.3
10	Lemons	2.4
11	Avocados	2.2
12	Nectarines	1.5
13	Cherries	1.3
14	Tangerines	1.3
15	Cranberries	0.9
16	Tangelos	0.6
17	Apricots	0.5
18	Limes	0.5

Data from USDA.

Figure 1.2: Rank order of USA fruit consumption, 1983 to 1984.

Ranking	Vegetable	Pounds per capita
1	Potatoes	77.7
2	Tomatoes	37.8
3	Lettuces	26.0
4	Onions	15.5
5	Sweet corn	14.7
6	Cucumbers and pickles	11.0
7	Carrots	9.4
8	Cabbage	9.0
9	Celery	7.5
10	Snap beans/French beans	7.4
11	Sweet potatoes	4.5
12	Peas	4.2
13	Broccoli	4.0
14	Bell peppers	3.2
15	Cauliflower	2.4
16	Spinach	1.3
17	Asparagus	0.7
18	Squash (winter)	0.6
19	Lima beans/butter beans	0.6

Data from USDA.

Figure 1.3: Rank order of USA vegetable consumption, 1983 to 1984.

Dietary Supplements

Beta-carotene is also available in supplement form. Supplements either contain synthetic (known as – all trans) beta-carotene, or 'natural' beta-carotene, made from two strains of the dunaliella alga (this contains a mixture of trans and cis – see Chapter 2).

The biggest suppliers of synthetic beta-carotene are Hoffmann-La Roche, the Swiss-based pharmaceuticals

Ranking	Fruit/vegetable	Pounds per capita	Mg of carotene per capita per year
1	Carrots	9.4	256.0
2	Sweet potatoes/yams	4.5	221.0
3	Tomatoes	37.8	85.8
4	Melons	20.2	62.2
5	Spinach	1.3	35.4
6	Lettuces	26.0	23.6
7	Sweet corn	14.7	16.0
8	Cabbage/sauerkraut	9.0	12.2
9	Broccoli	4.0	10.2
10	Peas	4.2	9.6
11	Oranges	29.7	6.7
12	Snap beans/French beans	7.4	4.7
13	Winter squash	0.6	4.6
14	Nectarines	1.5	3.4
15	Bananas	22.2	3.0
16	Bell peppers	3.2	2.9
17	Apricots	0.5	2.5
18	Apples	20.8	1.9

Data from USDA.

Figure 1.4: Contributions of fruits and vegetables to beta-carotene intake, 1983 to 1984 in the USA.

company, and BASF. Hoffmann-La Roche supply British brand leader VitaBrit; this supplement is also available as an algal-derived supplement. Several much smaller companies have sprung up recently and are manufacturing the 'natural' beta-carotene on algae farms.

The first commercial manufacture of beta-carotene was done by extracting beta-carotene from carrots, in the late 1950s.

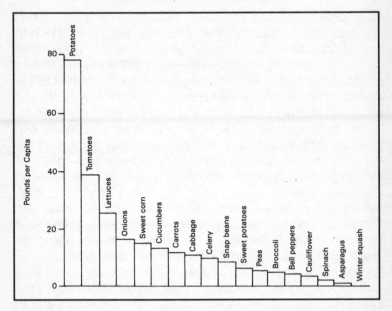

Figure 1.5: Vegetable consumption in the United States, 1983 to 1984 (in pounds per capita). (Data from USDA.)

Due to the unwieldy nature of such an operation, major production to vie with the synthetic manufacturers was not undertaken. Experiments with algae have been carried out since the early 1950s, and ideas on potential uses for large-scale culturing led on from those early experiments.

Beta-carotene from algae
Commercial attempts to make algae cultivation into an economic business were initiated at the end of the 1970s. There are now five main algae farms up and running: Koor-Foods in Israel, Microbio Resources in California, Cyanotech in Hawaii, Western Biotechnology, and Betatene, both in Australia. A role for the dunaliella alga was found in the business of beta-carotene supplementation. Dunaliella has since been described as 'the most successful microalga for outdoor cultivation.'[3]

Betatene won an Australian award in 1988 for developing a

new product within the food industry which had been commercially successful. Betatene was set up in 1985 to consolidate previous scientific work done on algal beta-carotene. The company's first full-scale plant was brought into production in April 1986 in Whyalla in South Australia. The plant is designed to process up to one million litres of brine per hour and to produce 20 tonnes of beta-carotene every year.

Two strains of dunaliella, namely *bardawil* and *salina*, can produce over 10 per cent of their own dry weight as beta-carotene; only one plant species produces more (the pheasant's eye narcissus mentioned in the Introduction). Dunaliella has no cell walls, which make it easily digestible when dried. Mass cultivation of algae normally requires lots of space for freshwater ponds, a temperate climate and year-round sunshine. Most of the areas of the world which suit these demands are arid environments with very salty seas.

Fortunately, the dunaliella alga thrives in these conditions and can happily live in seas containing more than 10 per cent salt. It is found in the Dead Sea in Israel, the Pink Lake in Australia and the Great Salt Lake in Utah, America. It is one of the very few microorganisms which can thrive in such a salty world.

The clumps of algae that can be seen in these lakes are often red in colour rather than green. This is because of the huge synthesis of beta-carotene by the cells to protect them from high intensity radiation from the sun. Strains of dunaliella which do not accumulate beta-carotene die when exposed to such high levels of natural light. Dunaliella bardawil contains equal amounts of the trans and cis forms of beta-carotene. Research into the effectiveness of cis in comparison with trans beta-carotene is controversial and is discussed in Chapter 3.

Commercial producers of dunaliella have developed special oblong ponds in which to grow the alga. Sunlight is absorbed by the algae which float in highly saline water; light is absorbed to a depth of just five centimetres, so the layer of algae is thin. The algae are continuously mixed to maintain even distribution of sunlight and to remove excess oxygen. Dunaliella is able to survive temperatures from below freezing to around 45°C, the optimal growth temperature is around 32°C. Harvesting is largely carried out using centrifuges, where the alga is whipped round at high speed and separated from water.

Methods have been developed to dehydrate wet dunaliella paste into dry dunaliella powder without damaging the beta-carotene. Antioxidants, such as vitamins C and E, are included to stop the beta-carotene from oxidizing and losing its potency.

The production of algal beta-carotene is more expensive than its synthetic counterpart – that's why supplements labelled 'natural' are more expensive. However, they are believed to be just as effective at converting to vitamin A and also act as antioxidants. Professor Ami Ben Amotz, based in Israel, has shown that adding beta-carotene rich algae to a vitamin A deficient chick increases levels of the vitamin. A similar response was also shown in vitamin A deficient rats.

VitaBrit provides 15 mg of the nutrient in each capsule. This dosage concurs with suggestions put forward by several scientists in the United Kingdom and the United States (see Chapter 10). Some recent studies have observed that beta-carotene absorption is greater from supplements than from foods. Below is a table showing the amounts of beta-carotene rich fruits or vegetables you would have to eat to obtain 15 mg of beta-carotene. Even with an equivalent measurement it is likely that not as much beta-carotene will be absorbed from food sources as from a concentrated supplement.

Food source	Carotene content mg per 110 g	Approximate daily amount to give 15 mg beta-carotene (lb)
Broccoli	1.9	2
Spinach	4.2	1
Carrots	7.3	0.5
Lettuces	0.8	5
Cucumbers	0.2	20
Watercress	2.7	1.5
Endives	0.4	10
Pumpkins	2.0	2
Tomatoes	0.8	5
Apricots	1.8	2
Plums	0.2	20
Peaches	0.4	10
Mangos	2.8	1.5
Bananas	0.2	18

Figure 1.6: Fruit and vegetable amounts needed to obtain 15 mg of beta-carotene.

Recipes Rich in Beta-Carotene

The following recipes are full of beta-carotene and will make an excellent regular addition to your diet.

Mango Breakfast Drink (Serves 2)
Beta-carotene content: 3 mg

Ingredients
450 ml skimmed milk
150 ml mango juice
5 tablespoons natural yogurt

Method
1. Put all the ingredients into the blender.
2. Blend until smooth. Pour into two large glasses and serve at once.

Watercress Soup (Serves 4)
Beta-carotene content: 8 mg

Ingredients
25 g butter
1 medium-sized onion
3 bunches watercress
25 g flour
1 litre vegetable stock
150 ml natural yogurt
salt and pepper to taste

Method
1. Finely chop onion and trim and chop watercress.
2. Heat the oil and fry the onion and watercress gently for 10 minutes over a low heat.
3. Add the stock and raise heat to moderate, stir constantly and add salt and pepper.
4. Once boiling, reduce heat and simmer for 15 minutes.
5. Liquidize in a blender until a purée.
6. Return to the pan and stir in the yogurt. Taste and adjust seasoning.
7. Reheat, then serve hot.

Spinach and Cheese Pancakes (Serves 4)
Beta-carotene content: 10 mg

Ingredients
Batter:
50 g wholemeal flour
50 g plain white flour
pinch salt
1 egg
300 ml skimmed milk

Filling:
25 g butter/margarine
25 g plain white flour
300 ml milk
225 g grated cheddar cheese
225 g frozen spinach
pinch of nutmeg

Method
Pancake:
1. Mix flours and salt in a bowl.
2. Make a well in the centre, add the egg and milk and gradually draw in the flour until a smooth batter is formed.
3. Beat well until smooth, cover and leave to stand for 30 minutes.
4. Heat a little oil in a 20 cm frying pan and pour in enough batter to cover the pan base.
5. Cook until the underside is golden, turn and cook the other side.
6. Place pancake on a plate, cover with greaseproof paper and repeat with remaining batter. You will be able to make about 12 pancakes.

Filling:
1. Put the butter, flour and milk in a pan. Heat gently, stirring all the time, until the butter melts. Bring to the boil and keep stirring for 2–3 minutes.

2. Add the cheese, spinach, nutmeg, salt and pepper to taste, stir until all the cheese has melted.
3. Divide the mixture between the pancakes. Roll up and put in a heatproof dish. Place under a hot grill for five minutes. Serve hot.

Carrot and Fruit Salad (Serves 4)
Beta-carotene content: 15 mg

Ingredients
4 medium carrots
1 eating apple
1 small orange
2 teaspoons lemon juice
150 ml natural yogurt
pinch of paprika
salt and pepper to taste
chopped parsley to garnish

Method
1. Peel and grate carrots. Peel and finely chop the apple and orange.
2. Combine with lemon juice in a large salad bowl.
3. Stir in salt, pepper and paprika to taste.
4. Pour the yogurt over the salad and garnish with parsley.

Carrot and Walnut Loaf
Beta-carotene content: 13 mg

Ingredients
75 g soft brown sugar
75 g butter or margarine
175 g carrots
1 teaspoon mixed spice
1½ tablespoons water
1 egg
75 g chopped walnuts
175 g self-raising wholemeal flour
pinch salt
1 tablespoon milk
walnut halves to decorate

Method
1. Peel and grate the carrots. Place in a bowl with butter, sugar, mixed spice and water.
2. Heat gently until sugar is dissolved then boil for three minutes stirring all the time.
3. Remove from heat and allow to cool.
4. Beat the egg and add to mix, along with the walnuts.
5. Stir in the flour, salt and milk. Mix well.
6. Set oven at 180°C/350°F/Gas Mark 4. Line and grease a 450 g loaf tin. Spoon in mix and bake in oven for one hour.
7. Remove from oven and cool for 10 minutes before turning out. Serve sliced with butter.

Apricot Fluff (Serves 4)
Beta-carotene content: 2 mg

Ingredients
100 g dried apricots
2 tablespoons water
3 tablespoons gelatine or agar agar
2 egg whites

Method
1. Soak apricots in water.
2. Cook in a little water until tender and then process in a blender.
3. Put the water in a heatproof container. Sprinkle in gelatine. Stand container in a pan of hot water and stir until gelatine dissolves.
4. Stir in apricot purée.
5. Whisk egg whites until stiff and gently fold in apricot mix.
6. Pour into four serving glasses and leave in fridge to set.
7. Serve with a crisp biscuit.

Notes

1. Heinonen, M.I., 'Carotenoids and provitamin A activity of carrot (Daucus carota L) cultivars', *Journal of Agricultural and Food Chemistry*, 1990, 38; pp. 609–42.
2. Micozzi, M.S., 'Carotenoid analyses of selected raw and cooked foods associated with a lower risk for cancer', *Journal of the National Cancer Institute*, 82, 4.
3. Ben-Amotz, A. and Avron, M., 'The biotechnology of mass culturing *dunaliella* for products of commercial interest', *Algal and Cyanobacterial Biotechnology*, (Cresswell R.C., *et. al.* eds.), Longman Scientific and Technical Press, 1989, pp. 90–114.

Chapter 2

The Structure of Beta-Carotene

Every single substance has its own identity of tiny atoms, a selection of components that make it totally individual. That's why oxygen is different from carbon dioxide, and coal different from gold. Beta-carotene is no exception. It has its own quota of atoms bonded together to make it a plant pigment, distinct from any other, distinguishable even from its close relatives in the carotenoid family. However, within each identity there can be different structures: the amount and type of atoms remains the same, but the pattern changes. These altered states are known as *isomers*, beta-carotene has two main isomers, called *trans* and *cis*.

When drawn as a chemical diagram (see Figure 2.1) the trans form is perfectly straight, whereas the cis form is bent. The difference is very subtle, but scientists are investigating the possibility that it may have an effect on the potency of beta-carotene. One could be better than the other, or perhaps they work best together.

Synthetic beta-carotene, which is found in many dietary supplements and in prescription medicines, usually consists of the all-trans form, because cis is very difficult to synthesize. In naturally occurring sources of beta-carotene, such as fruits and vegetables, cis and trans are found together. In all the human intervention trials so far established, synthetic beta-carotene has been used; as a result participants will have been absorbing beta-carotene in the trans state only.

The amount of cis beta-carotene contained in a fruit, vegetable or alga such as *Dunaliella* (see Chapter 2) depends on

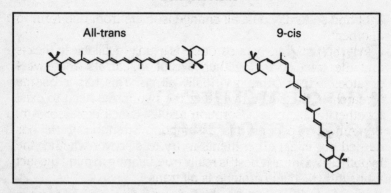

Figure 2.1: The chemical structure of trans and cis beta-carotene.

the intensity of sunlight during growth. Sun-exposed leaves, fruits and flowers contain up to 50 per cent cis beta-carotene, whereas carrots and sweet potatoes, which grow below the topsoil, contain very little.

A 1987 study found that fresh and processed fruits and vegetables contained between 1 and 29 per cent of the cis isomer.[1] Interestingly, a tinned carrot contains 20 times the amount of the cis isomer contained in a fresh carrot, the same with a canned sweet potato. Kale and spinach were the fresh vegetables with the highest proportions of cis – around 12 per cent – but canning a fruit or a vegetable allows the trans form of beta-carotene to change into cis.

Another paper reported that all fresh green vegetables contained between 19 and 28 per cent cis beta-carotene.[2] The alga dunaliella is comparatively high in cis beta-carotene, making up approximately half of the total beta-carotene content.

A 1988 study reported that 'heat processing' induced the formation of cis beta-carotene; the quantity formed was related to the intensity of the heat treatment, all treatments being over 100° centigrade.[3] This is the reason why canned vegetables contain so much more of the cis form than in their raw state – canning processes involve high temperatures to preserve the food. A study published in the early 1980s stated that heat, acid, light and solvents could all change isomers from one form to another.[4]

In its natural state beta-carotene is usually available in the cis and the trans form together, except in carrots and sweet potatoes, which contain virtually all cis. This has led some researchers to question whether the two forms need to exist together for the best absorption results. Israeli Professor Ami Ben-Amotz questions this assumption strenuously. He has carried out initial experiments to try to discover whether the hypothesis 'natural is best' is really true, bearing in mind the fact that synthetic beta-carotene is all trans.

Natural Beta-Carotene

The fact that algal beta-carotene contains equal amounts of cis and trans has always been a main selling point for its suppliers. They say that because it contains equal amounts of cis and trans it is better absorbed. The argument is that the cis form of beta-carotene is taken up more quickly by the lipids – fatty molecules – which carry it into the tissues. The synthetic trans beta-carotene is in crystal form, and takes the lipids longer to absorb. Even so, however, the longer time of absorption is probably only a matter of hours, and certainly not days.[5]

One of Professor Ben-Amotz's earlier papers examined whether chicks deficient in vitamin A could be supplemented with the beta-carotene rich alga *dunaliella bardawil*.[6] The study had a dual purpose, as alga is also a very good source of protein, which is a necessary additive in animal feed. Three groups of chicks were established: one group was fed a vitamin A deficient diet, the two others were given the same diet supplemented either with vitamin A, or with beta-carotene either from a synthetic source or from dry algae.

After five weeks, all the groups being supplemented were shown to have good vitamin A status. The chicks being supplemented with algal beta-carotene had similar growth patterns and weight gains to those supplemented with pure vitamin A; in appearance they had a more intense colour, and egg yolks also appeared brighter. Professor Ben-Amotz concluded by saying that *dunaliella bardawil* could be used as a practical source of vitamin A in the feed of poultry.

The experiment was repeated again in rat diets, and both the blood plasma and liver vitamin A concentration levels increased with supplementation.[7] However, the researchers found that the more beta-carotene was fed to the rats the less was converted to vitamin A; and this is consistent with other research (see Chapter 3).

Professor Ben-Amotz and his team published a later paper which reported that there was greater accumulation of cis beta-carotene than of trans in the livers of rats and chicks.[8] He wrote: 'Chicks and rats accumulate beta-carotene to a much greater extent when 9-cis beta-carotene is present in the diet.' In the liver of the chicks cis beta-carotene appeared to accumulate preferentially over trans; while in the rat liver the cis form stimulated the accumulation of cis and trans isomers. From these results Professor Ben-Amotz concluded that the cis isomer could serve as a good solvent for all-trans, either from the same capsule or in fruit and vegetables. He rounds off the paper by suggesting that the difference between cis and trans in his animal studies should be taken into account when 'higher levels of beta-carotene are desired to test its efficacy in other effects, such as the possible prevention of cancer'.

Since these two studies, Professor Ben-Amotz has been involved in studies looking into how people assimilate natural beta-carotene as opposed to the synthetic variety. Two studies have been established in Israeli hospitals. The first one at Tel-Hashomer is supplementing pre-operative patients with natural and synthetic beta-carotene. Thirty patients over 60-years-old will be supplemented with up to 20 mg of beta-carotene a day for two weeks before being operated on.

During the operation some arterial plaques will be removed for beta-carotene analysis (plaques contain lipids which are the main carriers of beta-carotene). The second study is based at Ramabm Hospital in Hypha, where a number of students will be taking high doses of natural and synthetic beta-carotene for one week. After that time their blood levels will be examined for beta-carotene levels.

More Initial Studies on Natural Beta-Carotene

As mentioned earlier, virtually all human intervention trials have used or are using synthetic beta-carotene capsules, rather than natural beta-carotene. Therefore scientists have not been able to ascertain whether the combination of the cis and trans isomers found in algae works better than the all-trans isomer found in synthetic beta-carotene. However two prominent studies using algal beta-carotene have been conducted using hamsters and mice. It is important to remember that rodents may differ from humans in their ability to absorb and process beta-carotene.

A study on hamsters showed that supplementation with algal beta-carotene stopped the development of mouth tumours, when the animals were subjected to treatment with a carcinogenic substance.[9] Groups of the animals were fed canthaxanthin, synthetic beta-carotene, mineral oil or nothing at all.

Those hamsters not receiving any supplement, or plain mineral oil, developed large tumours; those fed canthaxanthin developed very few; the synthetic beta-carotene animals presented some tumours, but they were smaller and on a lesser scale than the controls. In the hamsters given the algal beta-carotene no tumours whatsoever developed. A pre-cancerous condition did occur, but tumours did not result.

In the hamsters fed algal beta-carotene, microscopic changes called 'foci' did appear but, says the paper:

> they were being destroyed, probably by an immune response. These observations support the concept that the algae extract can prevent cancer development by stimulating an immune response to selectively destroy small initial foci of developing malignant cells.

The authors of the paper conclude:

> The effectiveness of the algae extract by oral administration in hamsters indicates that further research is warranted in

other species and other experimental tumour models. The chemoprevention of cancer may become a significant approach to the future management of cancer and micronutrients could possibly play a major role in cancer prevention.

The other study used mice to investigate the preventive role of algal beta-carotene in cases of mammary cancer.[10] A mainly Japanese research team was joined by Professor Ben-Amotz to carry out the experiment. The study, reported in 1989, concluded that the beta-carotene rich algae inhibited tumour growth through its conversion to vitamin A. The authors considered this interpretation of the results to be in line with a number of other studies, but added that experiments done by other researchers had found beta-carotene to have a role in cancer prevention independent from its capability to be converted into vitamin A.

Contrary Results

Not all the research done has shown natural beta-carotene, i.e. that containing the cis isomer, in such a good light. In 1944 a study showed that more vitamin A could be converted from all-trans beta-carotene than from cis beta-carotene in rats.[11] Another study, published in 1971, reported that processed yellow and green vegetables suffered a 15 to 35 per cent loss in vitamin A value due to the change from trans to cis isomers which happens during canning.[12]

A study further supporting the supremacy of trans beta-carotene over cis was published in 1987.[13] This used 16 healthy adults who had been on a low carotene diet for 10 days. The participants were six men and ten women between the ages of 18 and 60, and only people with non-deficient vitamin A levels were allowed into the study.

Participants in the study were given either 24 mg of algal beta-carotene a day, or just over 207.3 g of raw carrots (equivalent to 24 mg of beta-carotene), or placebo capsules. Treatment was spread over one week, and blood samples were collected before and after the treatment.

In the group taking the algal capsules, there was a pronounced shift in levels of cis and trans isomers in the blood. More trans than cis was measured, even though equal amounts of the two isomers had been consumed in the capsules. In the group consuming carrots there was a large increase in the level of the trans isomer, hardly surprising since carrots contain nearly all trans anyway, but what this did show was that trans beta-carotene could be absorbed intact through the gut.

The authors of the paper suggested several reasons for these results: first, cis beta-carotene passes unabsorbed through the gut; second, it is preferentially converted to vitamin A before the trans isomer; and third some cis isomers change to trans before they are absorbed. Professor Ben-Amotz has suggested that the cis isomers had already been absorbed by the lipids for transportation to tissues; this links with his theory that trans beta-carotene is badly absorbed by lipids (see page 37).

Research into the cis and trans forms of beta-carotene is a relatively minor part of the whole picture, but it is an interesting and potentially valuable one. More work needs to be done by a number of different scientists to gain a more objective appreciation of the situation. It is in the interests of the algae producers to be more favourable towards the cis form of beta-carotene, and the synthetic producers towards trans. Perhaps the next decade will shed more light on this hotly-contested question.

Notes

1. Quackenbush, F.W., *Journal of Liquid Chromatography*, 1987, 10(4), pp. 643–53.
2. Chandler, L.A. and Schwartz, S.J., *Journal of Food Science*, 1987, 52(3), pp. 669–72.
3. Chandler, L.A. and Schwartz, S.J., *Journal of Agriculture Food Chemistry*, 1988, 36, pp. 129–33.
4. Bauernfeind, J.C., *et al.*, 'Carotenes and vitamin A precursors in animal feed', in *Carotenoids as Colourants and Vitamin A Precursors: Technological and Nutritional Applications.*

Bauernfeind *et al* (eds.), Academic Press, New York, 1981, p. 563.

5. Ben-Amotz, A. *et al.*, Bioavailability of a natural isomer mixture as compared with synthetic all-trans beta-carotene in rats and chicks. *Journal of Nutrition*, 1989, 119, (7), pp. 1013–9.

6. Ben-Amotz, A. *et al.*, 'Use of the beta-carotene rich alga Dunaliella bardawil as a source of retinol', *British Poultry Science*, 1986, 27. pp. 613–19.

7. Ben-Amotz, A. *et al.*, 'The beta-carotene rich alga Dunaliella bardawil as a source of retinol in a rat diet', *British Journal of Nutrition*, 1988, 59. pp. 443–9.

8. Bauernfeind, *et al.*, op. cit.

9. Schwartz, J. *et al.*, 'Prevention of experimental oral cancer by extracts of Spirulina – Dunaliella algae', *Nutrition and Cancer*, 1988, 11(2). pp. 127–34.

10. Nagasawa, H. *et al.*, 'Inhibition by beta-carotene-rich algae dunaliella of spontaneous mammary tumourigenesis in mice', *Anticancer Research*, 1989, 9. pp. 71–6.

11. Deuel, H.J. *et al.*, 'Stereochemical configuration and provitamin A activity, I. All-trans beta-carotene and neo-beta-carotene', *Archive of Biochemistry and Biophysics*, 1944, 5, p. 107.

12. Sweeney, J.P. and Marsh, A.C., 'Effect of processing on provitamin A in vegetables', *Journal American Dietetics Association*, 1971, 59, p. 238.

13. Jensen, C.D. *et al.*, 'Observations on the effects of ingesting cis- and trans-beta-carotene isomers on human serum concentrations', *Nutrition Reports International*, 1987, 35(2). pp. 413–22.

Chapter 3

Intake and Absorption of Beta-Carotene

Dietary Intake of Beta-Carotene

Our dietary choice has never been wider, but the recently published *Dietary and Nutritional Survey of British Adults* has unearthed a worrying trend – young people are not eating as many nutritionally good foods as older generations.[1]

Out of groups of men and women aged 16 to 64, those between 16 and 24 years had the lowest daily intake of both vitamin A and beta-carotene, neither nutrient being able to make up for the shortfall left by the other. A low level of intake such as this will not cause deficiency diseases, but it does mean that the average member of this age group will gain only the bare minimum of benefit from this part of their diet.

The trend revealed by the survey is indicative of the popular teenage diet: fast foods, chips, burgers and crisps, sweets and snacks. These sorts of foods will meet protein requirements, but not supply the other essential nutrients and fibre found in fruits and vegetables, pulses and grains. The survey also revealed that people from lower socio-economic classes ate smaller amounts of food containing beta-carotene, lycopene, alpha-carotene, and cryptoxanthin.

Despite a trend towards convenience foods, vegetables (fresh, frozen and tinned) still account for around 70 per cent of beta-carotene consumed, with vegetables in meat products (pieces of carrot in a pasty, for example) being the second largest intake. Fruit only accounts for 3 per cent of beta-carotene intake in the United Kingdom.

Differences Between Men and Women

According to the *Dietary and Nutritional Survey of British Adults*, men have a higher daily intake of dietary carotenoids. However, research done by Dr David Thurnham at the Dunn Nutrition Centre in Cambridge has turned up some interesting results.

He and a colleague took measurements for five different carotenoids present in the blood of 2,000 British adults.[2] These consisted of three carotenoids which the body can convert into vitamin A – beta-carotene, cryptoxanthin and alpha-carotene – and two which it cannot – lutein and lycopene. The study found that men and women had similar blood measurements of lycopene and lutein; however when it compared the levels of beta-carotene, alpha-carotene and cryptoxanthin, women had higher measurements than men.

Thurnham concluded that men may have a greater need for vitamin A and will therefore convert more beta-carotene, alpha-carotene and cryptoxanthin into vitamin A, allowing less to go into the bloodstream as pure carotenoids. In order to match the female levels of beta-carotene, it seems men may have to eat even more foods containing this nutrient. Another study has recently confirmed that men have higher levels of vitamin A than women.[3] In addition to this, Thurnham's work showed that the quantities of beta-carotene measured in the blood increased with age, while lycopene decreased.

Dr Thurnham has investigated further the main factors responsible for determining plasma carotenes. He suggests that three factors influence the levels of the five main carotenoids in our blood. These are: dietary intake, age, and smoking. In the cases of beta-carotene, cryptoxanthin and alpha-carotene, dietary sources emerge as the major influence, followed by age. In the case of lycopene, the main factor is age; for lutein it is age and smoking.

This conclusion is borne out by the results of the official United Kingdom dietary survey, which showed that the older a person becomes the better their intake of carotenoids is. This trend is probably based on the rather ironic fact that, despite the health warnings about eating too much meat, older generations still stick to the 'meat and two veg' pattern, the 'two veg' giving them their increased levels of carotenoids. Conversely, younger people had higher levels of lycopene in their blood; this could be connected to their higher consumption of tomatoes and tomato products.

Another interesting dietary study was carried out by Dr Tom Sanders of Kings College London, who looked specifically at beta-carotene on its own (the Dietary Survey was based on all carotenoids).[5] Instead of looking at blood levels, he looked at dietary intake. The results showed that women consumed more beta-carotene daily than men. The average omnivorous man took in 1.4 mg, whereas the average omnivorous woman took in 3.8 mg. The highest intake for men was 7.8 mg, for women the amount was 8.8 mg.

Surprisingly, Dr Sanders showed that the average vegan fared little better considering their strict vegetarian diet. The male vegan consumed 2.4 mg every day, the female 4.7 mg. However, the highest daily consumption of beta-carotene was seen in vegans, the men reaching a staggering 21 mg, the women 12 mg. For comparison the doses used in current cancer intervention trials range from 15 mg to 50 mg, recommended intakes range from around 6 mg[5] to 15 mg.[6]

Comparison with the United States

In the United States the daily intake of beta-carotene is 1.5 milligrams, the most important source of beta-carotene is carrots, followed by sweet potatoes and tomatoes.[7] Cantaloup melon, spinach and lettuce are also good sources. Lettuce and tomatoes are not particularly good sources of beta-carotene, but if a lot of them are eaten over a year they do add up.

Many good sources of beta-carotene are hardly ever consumed in the United States. Winter squash, which has high levels of beta-carotene, is rarely eaten. Each person eats about 200 pounds of fruit every year, and again the most popular varieties, such as oranges, bananas and apples, have a very low beta-carotene content. Relying on dietary sources of beta-carotene means that if one does not like a certain type of food,

a major source of beta-carotene is often eliminated from the
diet.

Smoking and Beta-Carotene

Smoking is known to have an effect on the dietary intake of
certain foods. Smokers often eat 25 to 30 per cent less green
vegetables and fruit than non-smokers. In research studies
completed over the last twenty years a possible link has been
drawn between a greater risk of certain cancers, a low intake
of fruit and vegetables and low blood levels of beta-carotene.
One of the strongest correlations is for a protective effect of
beta-carotene against lung cancer.[8] Not only could smoking be
the main cause of lung cancer, it could reduce levels of beta-
carotene, which help to protect against lung cancer developing.

This hypothesis has generated a lot of interest, and there have
been several studies designed to see whether smoking actually
causes a reduction in levels, or whether the low levels are
caused by a diet lacking in foods containing beta-carotene.

In a study published in 1988 it was shown that men who
smoked one pack of cigarettes a day had over 25 per cent less
beta-carotene in their blood than non-smokers, despite a
similar dietary intake of beta-carotene containing foods.
Women had 20 per cent less in their blood than men. Similar
results were shown for alcohol consumption, men drinking 20
grammes of alcohol every day had 20 per cent less beta-
carotene in their blood, women 11 per cent less.[9]

Another study also showed significantly lower concentrations of beta-carotene in the blood among smokers and regular
alcohol drinkers. The intake of carotenoid-containing foods
was similar in these two groups, smokers and non-smokers.
Smokers who smoked more than 31 cigarettes every day and
who also drank regularly showed the lowest levels of beta-
carotene. Smoking and drinking seem to have a synergistic
effect on the lowering of levels. Another observation made in
the study was that the effect of lowering beta-carotene levels
was larger in drinking males than for smoking males. This was
not seen in women.[10]

A further study published in 1989 also demonstrated the negative effect of smoking on beta-carotene, but did not find a significant difference in the beta-carotene intake of smokers and non-smokers.[11] Smoking appears to have a general effect on the metabolism and even desire for types of food; one recent study showed that the dietary intake of carotenoids was lower in non-smokers exposed to passive smoke than it was in non-smokers not exposed to smoke.[12] Why it should deplete beta-carotene in particular (it does not deplete vitamin E) is as yet unknown; there are suggestions that it could activate enzymes which break it down, or it could provoke the body in some other way.

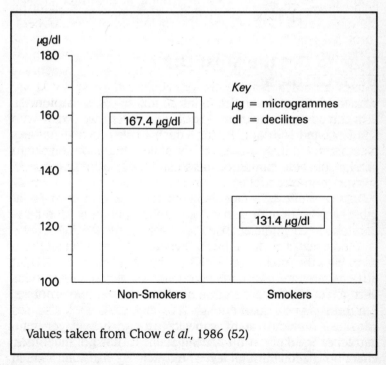

Figure 3.1: Smoking and plasma carotene levels.

Ultraviolet Light

There is some evidence that ultraviolet light can also deplete levels of carotenoids in the blood. A study completed by Dr Wendy White and colleagues showed that significant reductions occurred in both men and women after exposure to ultraviolet (UV) light over a two week period.[13] There was no reduction in vitamin A levels. Only one other study has been done on this subject to date, and no reduction was noticed.[14] Dr White writes that this may be due to lack of dietary controls (the subjects were allowed to eat anything they liked) and a smaller dose of UV light. The tentative conclusion of the White study is that reductions of circulating beta-carotene could increase the likelihood of a carcinogenic effect from UV light.

How to Get the Most Out of Beta-Carotene

With the factors of age, dietary intake and smoking to consider, how can we make the most of the beta-carotene we do eat? The US Food and Nutrition Board, which works out the nation's recommended daily amounts, has stated that about one-third of available beta-carotene is absorbed, and out of that, half is converted into retinol.

Beta-carotene is a fat-soluble nutrient; in other words fat must be present with beta-carotene if the optimum amount is to be absorbed. Sufficient bile flow is also needed to digest beta-carotene; bile is secreted by the liver to help digest fats, it also stimulates the production of certain digestive enzymes. Certain drugs can interfere with the production of bile, cholestyramine, used to reduce the absorption of cholesterol, is one example.

If there is not a good enough fat intake, deficiency diseases can occur. A study in an African village found that villagers who had a healthy diet of fruit and vegetables could not meet their vitamin A needs through it.[15] The deficiency had even caused blindness in some children. There was no point in increasing the amount of carotenoid-rich foods in the daily diet – the solution was to administer 18 grams of olive oil to the villagers every day. This guaranteed that the beta-carotene was being properly absorbed and converted.

Before you reel back in horror, and see your low fat diet going out of the window, take note that only a small amount of fat is needed to maximize the absorption of beta-carotene. For example you could eat chopped carrots in a stew containing a little oil. Or you could put some butter on your boiled carrots. If the carrots were served with a joint of meat or an oily fish such as mackerel, enough fat would be provided for the beta-carotene to be efficiently taken up.

In the current 'fat-free' climate, it may feel wrong to eat any fat with your food – but a little does help to mobilize beta-carotene. This is particularly important to remember if you are a vegan or vegetarian. Efficient transportation of vitamin A converted from beta-carotene also requires protein, or deficiency will occur. Non meat-eaters must ensure a good intake of alternative sources of protein, such as pulses. An adequate level of zinc is also needed for efficient conversion to vitamin A.

These principles apply to every other fruit and vegetable containing beta-carotene. Culinary preparation also has an effect on the bio-availability of beta-carotene, and should be taken into account. For example, chopped or puréed carrots have a much higher level of available beta-carotene; this is because plant cells have quite hard walls, which have to be broken down before letting out all the goodness; cooking begins to break the cell walls down and makes it easier to digest.

Surprisingly, tinned carrots have even higher quantities of beta-carotene available. It is possible to get as little as 1 per cent beta-carotene out of a raw carrot, so the message is: lightly cook your carrots, by steaming or in a little water. Overcooking can result in a severe decrease in bio-availability of carotenoids.

Blanching and freezing has little effect on beta-carotene content of a fruit or vegetable. However, because, in chemical terms, beta-carotene has numerous double bonds in its make-up, it is very susceptible to oxidation, a condition promoted by light, heat, metals and peroxides. On the whole, canning appears to enhance beta-carotene availability;

whereas drying techniques can lower concentrations.[16]

A healthy diet is a balanced diet, and consumption of other vitamins and nutrients is just as important. Beta-carotene is an antioxidant and can mop up free radicals (see Chapter 8), but it is protected from oxidation by vitamin E. Concentrating on one nutrient to the exclusion of all the others is not healthy – the benefits will be far greater if your overall vitamin, mineral and nutrient status is good.

Beta-Carotene from Supplement or Foods?

The US National Academy of Sciences has estimated that in comparison to pre-formed sources of vitamin A (such as liver and dairy products) the conversion of beta-carotene to vitamin A, weight for weight in food, is one-sixth. If beta-carotene is the only source of vitamin A, then dietary intake must be high in order to match it, and it is worth considering a supplement. Crystalline beta-carotene, found in many supplements, is almost totally absorbed, according to one study.[17]

A more recent piece of research compared the levels of seven carotenoids after ingesting either a beta-carotene capsule (all-trans) or a portion of vegetables with the same measurement of each carotenoid. The participants were fed for 11 days on a controlled low-carotenoid diet, and then split up into a pure beta-carotene group, and carrot, broccoli and tomato groups. None of the participants were smokers, and none took vitamin supplements or medication during the study.[18]

Figure 3.2 shows the amounts of vegetables needed to match the beta-carotene in a single supplement of either 12 mg or 30 mg, and how much of each carotenoid they had in them. A portion of carrots weighing 272 g is approximately the same as taking a 30 mg capsule of pure beta-carotene.

The researchers found that large, single intakes of carrots, broccoli and tomato juice, equivalent to 12 mg or 30 mg of pure beta-carotene, were unlikely to make much difference to normal blood levels of carotenoids:

The relatively poor plasma responses to a single, large portion of either cooked carrots, broccoli or canned tomato juice suggest that an individual's steady state carotenoid profile is a result of long-term dietary pattern and is little influenced by occasional large intakes of one food high in a particular carotenoid pigment.

Vegetable	Amount	Carotenoids	Level (mg)
Carrots	272 g	Beta-carotene	29
		Alpha-carotene	9
Broccoli	600 g	Lutein	5
		Beta-carotene	6
Tomato juice	180 g	Lycopene	12
Beta-carotene	Capsule	Beta-carotene	12
Beta-carotene	Capsule	Beta-carotene	30

Figure 3.2: Beta-carotene comparison between vegetables and capsules.

The study found that people eating an equivalent amount of carrots to 12 mg and 30 mg beta-carotene capsules only absorbed one-fifth and one-third respectively of that absorbed by those taking capsules alone. It also showed that a 30 mg capsule was not two-and-a-half times better absorbed than a 12 mg capsule – it was only one-and-a-half times better. This result indicates that elevated beta-carotene levels are not the necessary outcome of taking a high-dose capsule; it may be more economical to stick to a low-dose one.

This study shows that maintaining a consistent and regular pattern of eating beta-carotene – either from food sources or as a supplement such as VitaBrit – and other carotenoids is more beneficial than consuming one-off boosters. The researchers were also able to identify participants who were consistently poor absorbers, this illustrates the variation in individuals and shows that blood levels of carotenoids do not necessarily show an accurate picture of dietary intake.

Another group of scientists carried out a study to examine how beta-carotene was absorbed by humans. The team looked first at the uptake of beta- and alpha-carotene from raw carrot, and compared it to a placebo. They found that blood levels of the two carotenes peaked about five hours after ingestion of the carrots.[19] In another study the same team also showed that blood levels of beta-carotene rose higher through the ingestion of supplements, rather than raw carrots.[20]

From these studies we can see that a supplement is much more effective than a selection of vegetables rich in beta-carotene at raising blood levels. A background intake of vegetables and fruit rich in carotenoids will help to establish steady tissue levels. A supplement may be advisable if a person is unable to eat the appropriate fruit and vegetables every day.

Individual Considerations

It has been established that the absorption of beta-carotene from a supplement is higher than that from a piece of fruit or a vegetable. Still, some people taking supplements simply do not absorb beta-carotene as well as others – effective absorption remains at the mercy of a body's make-up. Research published in 1988 underlined this variation.[9] The administration of beta-carotene produced a great deal of variation of plasma levels. There is no single explanation why bioavailability of beta-carotene shows such individual variations.' (There was no danger of any of the participants in the study not taking their daily capsules, because dosage was overseen.)[21]

The study found that daily administration of 15 mg of beta-carotene over eight weeks resulted in significant increases in blood levels; these levels returned to normal between 10 and 30 days after the use of beta-carotene was discontinued. Administration of 45 mg daily for four weeks resulted in elevated levels after just four days of treatment. Levels returned to normal after 10 to 40 days.

As has been discussed, a little fat aids the absorption of beta-carotene, and this study also contained a section designed to test this out. Participants were obliged to take 45 mg of beta-carotene for three weeks, and either be put on a high-fat or low-fat diet for the first five days. Those on the high-fat diet reached very high blood levels during the first five days, after that time they were allowed to eat whatever kinds of food they wanted, but beta-carotene levels remained steady. After discontinuation, beta-carotene levels declined gradually.

The low-fat group showed elevated levels of beta-carotene in the blood, but not until 15 days of the treatment had gone by. Levels went back to normal between 7 and 23 days after treatment had been stopped.

In addition to studying the effects of daily dosage and the consumption of fat, the research team also looked at whether intermittent doses of beta-carotene could raise levels of beta-carotene in the blood. Doses of 45 mg every five days were given and a steady elevation of beta-carotene levels was observed. One participant stayed on the dose for eight weeks – and maintained the level within a small range of deviation. A similar dose given at intervals longer than five days was not as effective, and was unable to sustain levels at a steady standard.

Conclusion

As beta-carotene is not considered a vitamin, it has no official recommended daily amount (RDA). However, it is a very important safe source of vitamin A and should not be forgotten about. If there proves to be a positive association between protection against certain cancers and beta-carotene (see Chapter 6 and 7), then official nutrition bodies may be prepared to give it an RDA. Until that time, intake can only be judged by scientists in the field (see Chapter 10).

Increasing your intake of fruits and vegetables rich in beta-carotene and other carotenoids can do nothing but good, and should be part of a healthy diet anyway. The decision of whether to take a supplement is an entirely personal one; but it will provide a much more consistent source of beta-carotene, and you don't have to chomp your way through pounds of fruit and vegetables every day to get it – a very useful thing if your diet is lacking animal sources of vitamin A.

Notes

1. Gregory, J., et al., *The Dietary and Nutritional Survey of British adults*, HMSO, Social Survey Division, London 1990.
2. Thurnham, D.I., 'Do higher vitamin A requirements in men explain the difference between the sexes in plasma provitamin A carotenoids and retinol?' *Proceedings of Nutrition Society*, 1988, 47, p. 181A.
3. Nierenberg, D.W. *et al.*, 'Determinants of plasma levels of beta-carotene and retinol', *American Journal of Epidemiology*, 130, 3, pp. 511–21.
4. Sanders, T. and Key, *Human Nutrition: Applied Nutrition*, 1987, 41A, pp. 204–11.
5. Lachance, P., 'Dietary intake of carotenes and the carotene gap', *Clinical Nutrition*, vol. 7, 3, May/June 1988.
6. Diplock, A.T., 'Dietary supplementation with antioxidants: Is there a case for exceeding the recommended dietary allowance?' *Free Radical Biology and Medicine*, 1987, vol. 3, pp. 199–201.
7. See 5.
8. Ziegler, R.G., 'A review of epidemiologic evidence that carotenoids reduce the risk of cancer', *American Journal of Nutrition*, 119, (1), pp. 116–22.
9. Stryker, W.S. *et al.*, 'The relation of diet, cigarette smoking, and alcohol consumption to plasma beta-carotene and alpha tocopherol levels', *American Journal of Epidemiology*, vol. 127, 2, pp. 293–96.
10. Aoki, K. *et al.*, 'Smoking, alcohol drinking and serum carotenoid levels', *Japanese Journal of Cancer Research*, (Gann), 1987 (Oct), 78, pp. 1049–56.
11. Nierenberg, D.W. *et al.*, 'Determinants of plasma levels of beta-carotene and retinol', *American Journal of Epidemiology*, 130, 3, pp. 511–21.
12. Sidney, S. *et al.*, *American Journal of Epidemiology*, 1989, 129, pp. 1305–9.
13. White, W.S. *et al.*, 'Ultraviolet light-induced reductions in plasma carotenoid levels', *American Journal of Clinical Nutrition*, 1988, 47, pp. 879–83.

14. Berne, B. *et al.*, 'UV treatment of uraemic pruritus reduces the vitamin A content of the skin', *European Journal of Clinical Investigation*, 1984, 14, pp. 203–6.

15. Roels, O.A. *et al.*, 'Carotene balances in boys in Ruanda where vitamin A deficiency is prevalent', *Journal of Nutrition*, 1958a, 65, pp. 115–27.

16. Erdman, J., 'Factors affecting the biochemistry of vitamin A, carotenoids and vitamin E', *Food Technology*, 1988, 42, no. 10, pp. 214–16, 219–21.

17. Borenstein, B. and Gordon, H.T., 'Addition of vitamins, minerals and amino acids to foods', in *Karmas and Harris*, 1988, p. 609.

18. Brown, E.D. *et al.*, 'Plasma carotenoids in normal men after a single ingestion of vegetables or purified beta-carotene', *American Journal of Clinical Nutrition*, 1989, 49, pp. 1258–65.

19. Jensen, *et al.*, 'Acute effects of dietary carotenes on serum alpha- or beta-carotenes in humans', *Nutrition Reports International*, 1986, 33, pp. 117–22.

20. Jensen, *et al.*, 'Repletion and depletion of serum alpha- and beta-carotene in humans with carrots and an algae-derived supplement', *Acta Vitaminologica et Enzymologica*, 1985, 7, pp. 187–98.

21. Dimitrov, N.V., 'Bioavailability of beta-carotene in humans', *American Journal of Clinical Nutrition*, 1988, 48, pp. 298–304.

Chapter 4

Beta-Carotene –
A Safe Nutrient

A Safe Source of Vitamin A

Vitamins are 'essential for the life and well-being of animals and man'.[1] We cannot manufacture vitamins inside our bodies, so we have to consume them through our diets. The main vitamins are A, B group, C, D and E, and all are available in different foods. For example, vitamin A is in liver and dairy produce, and vitamin C is in most fruit and vegetables, particularly currants and rosehips.

Each vitamin has been given an official recommended daily amount (RDA) to try to ensure that no one becomes deficient in any of these vital nutrients. Deficiency diseases are generally rare in Western nations, but they do still occur in the Third World, where food supply and variety can be extremely limited.

It is the people in the Third World in particular who rely heavily on the beta-carotene found in fruit and vegetables. This is because beta-carotene can be converted to vitamin A if there is a shortage from other sources. Approximately fifty different carotenoids have the ability to form vitamin A, but beta-carotene is by far superior to the others; from each of its molecules it can make two molecules of vitamin A – a unique characteristic. For many people, including Third World populations, and vegans and lacto-vegetarians in the West, beta-carotene is the main – often only – source of vitamin A. It is a very valuable nutrient, of which many people are not even aware.

The Conversion of Beta-Carotene

Vitamin A derived from animal sources is called pre-formed vitamin A; this is because it does not have to undergo any kind of conversion once inside the digestive system. Beta-carotene is called a pro-vitamin A, because it needs to be converted inside the gut before it can be used as vitamin A.

Vitamin A is vital for human health; deficiency can result in a hardening of the skin and mucous membranes, leading to severe dryness and night blindness. It contributes to the general health of the eyes, the skin, hair, teeth and gums, builds resistance to respiratory infections, and is an important element in the control of cell proliferation.

Once converted, beta-carotene can do just the same things as vitamin A. The main difference between the two types is toxicity; because vitamin A is fat-soluble it is not excreted through the urine, and this means that it concentrates in body tissues and organs, and can cause ill-health.

If pre-formed vitamin A (from animal sources) is ingested in too high a quantity, it can induce a physical state of hypervitaminosis A, and the body begins to show signs of ill-health. A study in 1980 recorded up to 600 cases of hypervitaminosis A, with symptoms including peeling and redness of the skin, disturbed hair growth, loss of appetite, and sickness.[2] Most of these symptoms disappeared as soon as the person cut down intake of vitamin A.

Severe overdosing on vitamin A can cause liver damage, because vitamin A concentrates in the liver. A few people have died of hypervitaminosis A. Arctic explorers have died from eating polar bear liver and seal liver. These wild animals have extremely high concentrations of vitamin A in their livers. There are also reports that vitamin A is a teratogen (causes defects in the foetus) – but this is still a controversial issue, and research is ongoing.

Beta-Carotene, Not Toxic

Beta-carotene has none of these potential toxic effects. If the body is low in vitamin A supplies, it will convert beta-carotene, but as soon as it has been topped up the conversion stops. The better the vitamin A status, the less beta-carotene is converted. Any beta-carotene not converted is simply stored in the fatty tissues or passed out.

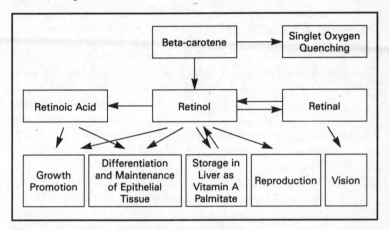

Figure 4.1: The various forms of vitamin A and their biological roles.

Administration of high doses of beta-carotene cannot lead to hypervitaminosis A. If you want to take a self-administered vitamin A supplement, then it is much safer to take a beta-carotene supplement (such as VitaBrit) which will only give you as much of the vitamin as your body needs.

There is only one known side-effect of taking beta-carotene in food or supplement form and most people seem to like it! The condition stems from hypercarotenemia, i.e. high levels of beta-carotene in the blood, and is called hypercarotenodermia, a yellowing of the skin which resembles a light tan. A yellow tinge on the palms of the hands and the soles of the feet will be noticeable if a person is consuming over 30 milligrams of beta-carotene a day.[3]

If a person is on very high doses, during the treatment of a light sensitive condition for example, then the whole of the skin will take on a faintly tanned look – gaining a healthy colour without frazzling in the sun! Hypercarotenodermia disappears when the source of beta-carotene is cut off. Sometimes the condition appears in infants fed processed foods containing a lot of finely ground carrots.[4]

Used in Clinical Trials

Over the last fifteen years the increasing number of studies linking beta-carotene with reduced rates of certain cancers (see Chapter 7) have caused a huge surge of interest in this simple plant pigment. This has resulted in the initiation of over seven intervention studies to look at the effects of beta-carotene. An intervention trial is the most influential stage of research, when people are supplemented with a substance to see whether it can influence the development of certain diseases.

There are no worries about safety when supplementing people with beta-carotene. The American National Cancer Institute is funding seven intervention trials on beta-carotene, and supplementation with the nutrient ranges from 15 mg to 50 mg on a daily basis. This is up to 30 times the usual intake level. In theory 30 mg of beta-carotene could be converted to 50,000 international units (IU) of vitamin A (the recommended daily amount is 10,000 IU). However this would only happen if the body needed that amount of vitamin A, otherwise it would stay uncoverted.

Long-term supplementation with beta-carotene has already occurred, with no adverse results. A pilot study to investigate the links between beta-carotene and lung cancer was established by Dr Joseph Constantino at the University of Pittsburgh, Philadelphia. For one year a group of 300 men received 15 mg daily of beta-carotene. This dose produced a ten-fold increase of levels of beta-carotene in the blood, with no toxic side-effects and no significant yellowing of the skin.[5]

Sun Sensitivity

The most reliable source of information on the safety of beta-carotene comes from its use as a treatment for people with light sensitivity conditions, in particular the congenital defect erythropoietic protoporphyria (EPP), when sufferers are sensitive to visible light, made worse on a sunny day. Sufferers usually develop it in childhood, sometimes in early infancy, and it manifests itself as a burning sensation on the skin, followed by skin reddening, itching and swelling.

The observation of plant biology played a crucial role in the discovery that long-term supplementation with beta-carotene could help EPP and related conditions. Researchers saw that carotenoids in plants played an important protective role against chlorophyll photosenitization. Chlorophyll enables a plant to manufacture energy from the sun; consequently it is very sensitive to light. However, without substances such as beta-carotene to absorb the reactive energy molecules produced by excess radiation, the plant would become over-sensitive to light and would burn up.

Professor Micheline Mathews-Roth, of Harvard Medical School, has spent over twenty years studying the effects of beta-carotene on EPP and related conditions. The strength of the plant evidence convinced her to test out beta-carotene on EPP sufferers.[6]

Preliminary experiments in 1961 had suggested that the onset of the skin reddening caused by light sensitivity could be delayed by administration of beta-carotene. In 1969 Professor Mathews-Roth decided to try out her hypothesis on humans. Between 1969 and 1975, 133 patients suffering from EPP were treated with beta-carotene.

Almost all the patients had to wear protective clothing when in the sun, some suffered during the winter too, and their activities were severely limited by EPP. During the period of the study, the professor and her fellow researchers worked out a series of dosages for beta-carotene still recommended for use today.

The doses begin at 60 milligrams per day for children aged between 1 and 4 years, to the top dose of over 180 mg daily for those patients over 16. The dose is administered over four to six weeks and the patient is asked not to increase their exposure to the sun until some yellow discolouration has appeared on the palms of the hands (hypercarotenodermia).

Once the yellowing is noticeable, the patient can gradually increase time spent in the sunlight. As soon as the symptoms start to reappear, sufferers know the maximum time their skin can tolerate being in the sun. The dosage of beta-carotene can be increased up to a total of 300 mg for those over 16 years old. If the treatment at these high levels has no effect after three months duration then, says Professor Mathews-Roth, 'It can be assumed that beta-carotene therapy will not be effective for that patient, and the medication should be discontinued.'

In 1975, at the end of the study, the United States Food and Drug Administration (FDA) approved the use of beta-carotene for the treatment of EPP. Mathews-Roth and her colleagues found that 84 per cent of the patients treated increased by a factor of three or more their ability to tolerate sunlight exposure without experiencing the symptoms of EPP; there were no abnormally high levels of vitamin A measured in the blood, and no signs of hypervitaminosis A.

On average, it took between one and two months before an increased tolerance was noticed, after which point most of the patients were able to spend much more time outdoors. The children involved in the trial were able to play outside with their friends – a real novelty for them.

Many of the older patients recorded that they were able to develop a suntan for the first time in their lives; before the treatment they could not tolerate the sun for long enough periods. Professor Mathews-Roth writes:

> It was the impression of several of the patients that the acquisition of the tan, plus the beta-carotene, added to their protection from the sun's effects. The majority of the patients noted that when they are taking beta-carotene, those reactions from the sun that do occur are less severe in intensity and duration than before therapy ... No serious side effects from beta-carotene have been reported.

In the paper which summarizes this information, 22 separate studies are cited which have also shown a beneficial effect using beta-carotene on EPP sufferers.[7] The authors emphasize that the treatment must be tailored for each individual, increasing the dose until the right level is found.

Beta-carotene supplementation has also been tried out with varying degrees of success on Gunther's disease, polymorphous light eruption, actinic reticuloid, solar urticaria, hydroa aestivale, hydroa vacciniforme and porphyria variegata. However, treatment of EPP remains the most successful. Beta-carotene preparations are now available as prescription products, such as Solatene.

Suntanning

After the success of the EPP trial, Professor Mathews-Roth decided to carry out a controlled trial to see whether beta-carotene altered the response of fair-skinned people to sunlight.[8] The study found that high doses of beta-carotene had a small but significant effect in increasing the amount of time that could be spent in the sun before the skin reddened. But the Professor writes, 'The observed effects were too small to recommend the use of beta-carotene as a protective agent for sunburn.'

Curiously, the people in the study developed a better tan than those in the placebo group. This finding concurs with two other similar observations made in the 1920s and 1930s: one found that hypercarotenemia made tanning easier;[9] the other that carotenemia in tubercular children prevented sunburn.[10] Today, you can buy special 'tanning' preparations containing beta-carotene; they may well have a protective effect, but much more work needs to be done to prove this is so. Meanwhile, the best antidote to the ravages of the sun is to lard on the factor 15 and avoid baking on the beach.

Method of Action

The factor behind beta-carotene's beneficial effect is believed to be its ability to quench highly reactive singlet oxygen (see Chapter 8). Various studies have suggested that carotenoids can quench free radicals and singlet oxygen generated during exposure to UV light.[11,12,13] UV light is responsible for many skin conditions, including skin cancers and malignant melanoma.[14] However the mechanisms of action still need to be researched further before a conclusion can be reached on whether beta-carotene can protect against these types of cancer.

Safety as an Additive and Food Supplement

Since the 1950s, beta-carotene has been produced as a food additive to give products an orange/yellow colour. Pure, crystalline beta-carotene has been approved by the US Food and Drug Administration as a colour additive for use in foods, drugs and cosmetics. It also has 'GRAS' (generally recognized as safe) status relating to its use as a supplement. It can be found in many different food types, ranging from cereals to fruit squashes. Beta-carotene is often used as a 'natural' alternative to the coal-tar based 'azo' dyes. The US ADI (acceptable daily intake) for beta-carotene as a food additive is 5 milligrams per kilogram of body weight.

Other Worries Unfounded

Concerns have been raised that high levels of beta-carotene could lower the white blood cell count, disturb the menstrual cycle, cause damage to the foetus and produce crystal deposits in the retina. None of these challenges to the safety of beta-carotene stand up against the evidence as presented by beta-carotene expert Dr Adrianne Bendich in a recent review.[15] Professor Mathews-Roth did not find any lowering of the white blood cell count in EPP patients taking high doses of beta-carotene over five years. Neither did she find any evidence of abnormalities in the babies of women who were taking high doses of beta-carotene as treatment for photosensitivity conditions, or in women who were hypercarotenemic during pregnancy and who consumed a large amount of food containing beta-carotene. She did not observe any menstrual disruption in women taking 180 mg of beta-carotene daily.

In addition, another researcher found no difference in the

carotene intake or blood levels of beta-carotene in female runners with normal and abnormal menstrual cycles.[16] An examination of the retinas of 26 different people with EPP, treated with high doses of beta-carotene for up to ten years, showed no signs of crystal deposits.[17]

The evidence in favour of beta-carotene's safety is overwhelming. Observations made by Professor Mathews-Roth and colleagues have been invaluable. They have shown that daily supplementation over 15 years with extremely high doses of beta-carotene 60 times the normal intake have no ill-effects except for yellowing of the skin, a condition which is completely reversible if supplementation is discontinued. Whether beta-carotene is used to treat light-sensitive conditions, as a food additive, or as an alternative to vitamin A, its safety record is impeccable.

Notes

1. Marks, J., *The vitamins: their role in medical practice*. MTP Press, Lancaster, 1988.
2. Bauernfeind, J.C., *The safe use of vitamin A. A report of the international vitamin A consultative groups (IVACC)*, The Nutrition Foundation, Washington, 1980.
3. Bendich, A., 'The safety of beta-carotene', *Nutrition and Cancer*, 1988, 2, pp. 207–14.
4. Lascari, A.D., 'Carotenemia: a review', *Clinical Pediatrics*, 20, 1981, pp. 25–9.
5. *ibid*.
6. Mathews-Roth, M.M., 'Beta-carotene therapy for erythropoietic protoporphyria and other photosensitivity diseases', *Biochemie*, 68, 1986, pp. 875–84.
7. *ibid*.
8. Mathews-Roth, M.M. *et al.*, *Journal of Investigative Dermatology*, 1972, 59, pp. 349–53.
9. Sandler, A.S., *Archivos de Pediatria*, 1935, 52, pp. 391–406.
10. Bendes, J.H., *Minnesota Medicine*, 1926, 9, pp. 112–14.
11. Dubertret, L. *et al.*, *Photochemistry and Photobiology*, 1982, 35, pp. 103–7.

12. Mathews-Roth, M.M., *Photochemistry and Photobiology*, 1984, 40, pp. 63–7.
13. Mathews-Roth, M.M., *Photochemistry and Photobiology*, 1986, 43, pp. 91-3.
14. Bolger, J. *et al.*, 'Sunscreens: efficacy, use and misuse', *Southern Medical Journal*, 77, 11, pp. 1421–27.
15. Constantino, P. *et al.*, 'Serum levels after administration of a pharmacologic dose of beta-carotene', *American Journal of Clinical Nutrition*, 1988, 48, pp. 1277–83.
16. Richards, S.R. *et al.*, 'Serum carotene levels in female long-distance runners', *Fertility and Sterility*, 43, 1985, pp. 79–81.
17. Poh-Fitzpatrick, M.B. *et al.*, 'Absence of crystalline retinopathy after long-term therapy with beta-carotene', *Journal of the American Academy of Dermatology*, 11, 1984, pp. 111–13.

Chapter 5

A Look at Cancer

In the previous chapter we have read that beta-carotene is a valuable, safe source of vitamin A and is used successfully in the treatment of light-sensitive conditions. In addition to these two well-known roles of this nutrient is a possible third: research over the last twenty years indicates that it could protect against certain types of cancer. Before taking a look at the evidence, it may be useful to have a greater understanding of the nature of cancer and its causes.

Next to heart disease, cancer is Britain's biggest killer, said by the Cancer Research Campaign to affect one in three people. Despite over fifty years of serious research there is still no cure – perhaps there never will be. Why does cancer remain such an enigma? Surely if science can devise ways to replace whole organs it can cope with cancer?

The answer is plain and simple – cancer is one of the most complex diseases ever to stretch the imagination of scientists. There are over 200 types, many with different causes, manifestations and predicted outcomes (or prognoses). As top academic Richard Peto wrote:

> It makes as little sense to lump together cancers of the lung, stomach and intestine when considering the causes of cancer as to lump together cholera, tuberculosis and syphilis.[1]

His words are echoed by many others in the field; different cancers must be treated individually. Their effects on human beings are also very individual – some people manage to shake cancer off, while others don't. Everyone seems to have a relative who smoked 60 cigarettes a day, did no exercise and still managed to live until they were 90. There are always exceptions to the rule.

Extensive research has shown that cancer is a multi-stage disease, influenced by many factors. It is extremely difficult to isolate one specific factor and say 'that is the cause.' In the words of Elizabeth Skinner from the British Cancer Research Campaign, the disease is a 'whole story': a story of external influences, internal health and genetic susceptibility, and there are many different versions of the story.

What is certain is that cancer is killing far too many people and there is no immediate 'cure ' – even cancer patients who are cured from the disease have to undergo further sessions of treatment, sometimes long-term. Unable to find one solid factor that works against all cancers, research work has blossomed into the area of prevention. The experts want to stop cancer before it has even started.

The Initiation of Cancer

All cancers are caused by genetic mutation; the mutation begins in one cell or a group of cells, the tiny building bricks which make up our bodies. We are each made up of billions of cells and each one contains the genetic substance DNA – a blueprint for living – which instructs a cell what to do. Some may build bone, some store fat and some make up blood. Whatever their job, in order to function properly the DNA must be kept in an unaltered form.

One modern theory is that the cells inside our bodies are frequently under attack from various hostile substances. Normally our internal defences such as white blood cells and macrophages (scavenging cells) stop these substances from harming us. They patrol the tissues and bloodstream looking for any 'foreigners' that they do not recognize; if they do find anything strange the intruders are swiftly disposed of or quenched. If a hostile substance does manage to avoid these defences and damage a cell's DNA, then there are busy 'repair' proteins – the second line of defence – which will chop out the offending part of the cell, leaving the rest unimpaired.

Normally, our defences are enough, but sometimes the routine goes wrong. For example a cancer-causing substance (carcinogen) could side-step the defences and manage permanently to damage DNA. Or a highly reactive free radical such as the hydroxyl radical (see Chapter 8) could severely disable a cell, leaving it mutated. Turning to genetic factors, it is quite possible that a certain gene in a cell will be born, as it were, with the ability to trigger cancer. The effects of viruses are strongly linked to some cancers; the estimate made by Dr Richard Peto is that up to 10 per cent of cancers could be caused by a virus. The hepatitis-B virus is known to be a cause of liver cancer, there are also some leukaemia viruses; cancers of the cervix, penis, vulva and anus may have viral causes too – scientists are investigating.

What Happens After the Mutation?

It is believed that all cancers have several stages, the most important ones being initiation – when a cell is first damaged – promotion – when the cell is influenced by other carcinogenic factors – and proliferation – when the cell or group of cells actively mutates to cause a tumour.

It all sounds very neat and logical, but there is no hard and fast rule about how long it will take for a cancer to show itself. Once a cell's DNA has mutated it can become cancerous then and there, or it can lie dormant to be triggered by something else later. Some carcinogens can cause damage to DNA in the initial process – these are called 'mutagens'; other carcinogens do not have the ability to be mutagens, but can act as trigger factors to the already damaged cell later on in the promotion stage.

So what actually happens to the mutant cell? Normally, most cells have the ability to reproduce and regenerate themselves when necessary – we only have to look at how we shed our outer layer of skin to understand that – but when a mutant cell is triggered off, it begins to reproduce itself uncontrollably. The DNA which usually tells it not to is no longer functioning as it should; it is as though the DNA has suffered shellshock, rather than being killed.

And so begins a treacherous progression that causes a tumour to grow and spread. The mutant cells use up nutrients just like the healthy cells, but serve no purpose – they simply replicate over and over again. After billions of similarly damaged cells have replicated themselves, a tumour or lesion can be detected. The detection will be much easier in external cancers such as breast and skin which can be felt and seen; internal cancers are much more difficult to pinpoint.

Eventually there are so many mutant cells that they outnumber the healthy cells and can spread to other parts of the body through the bloodstream and lymph (tissue fluid), where they metastasize (form secondary cancers). It only takes one tiny cell to break off and travel along the bloodstream to form another tumour. Secondaries themselves can take up to five years to grow and it is at this stage that cancer is particularly dangerous, the primary site may have been successfully treated but a secondary cancer could crop up anywhere else in the body up to five years after the initial treatment.

How Can Cancer be Detected?

One of the most perplexing aspects of cancer is that without being screened you cannot tell whether you have the disease until you get symptoms, and screening only exists for a few cancers, such as breast and cervix. By the time one can physically feel that there is something wrong, it is often very hard to stop the cancer's steady march.

The reason why lung, stomach and pancreas cancers have such poor prognoses is that they often spread without symptoms – because they are internal and you can't see or feel them until it's too late. Another factor which affects the seriousness of a cancer is whether it is in an area of fast-flowing circulation. Cancers near to a very busy area – such as the neck – will grow much more rapidly, whereas cancers in low blood-flow locations – such as the spine – will grow slowly and have little opportunity to break off and form secondary tumours. There is no definitive time over which a malignant cancer can develop; from initiation to promotion can take up to thirty years.

Despite millions of pounds being poured into cancer research, the best-known cure for cancer remains surgery, followed by killing the cancer cells via chemotherapy (drugs) or radiotherapy (radiation). If a cancer has already spread to other parts of the body, total success with such methods may be more difficult to achieve.

Technically speaking, all cancers are treatable, but some respond better than others. For example in the United Kingdom there is a 97 per cent survival rate for skin cancers (excluding melanoma), a 70 per cent survival rate for cancer of the uterus and a 62 per cent survival rate for bladder cancer. If breast cancer is detected early on, the five year survival rate after diagnosis is 80 per cent. The story for lung, stomach and pancreas is very different. Stomach has the lowest survival rate of just 11 per cent.

The Profile of Cancer

Cancer is not a new disease, nor is it a disease confined to Western nations. Its incidence is spread across many centuries and spans the world. There is evidence of bone cancer in dinosaur skeletons, and cancers have been found in Egyptian mummies. It was the Greek doctor Hippocrates who first gave cancer a name, he called it *karkinoma*, which means 'crab' – he noticed that some growths had a crab-like appearance. The word *cancer* is latin for crab and is the term we now use.

Cancer research has taken on huge proportions, probably because other life-threatening diseases such as tuberculosis and polio have been virtually wiped out. In the United States in 1971 Congress passed the National Cancer Act, and war on cancer was declared. US statistics show that in people of 45 years and over, there has been very little change in the death rate from cancer in the last 35 years. The disease is so widespread that virtually every country in the world either runs a cancer-based charity, or has a Government institute to look into the subject.

ALL CANCERS				100%

MEN		WOMEN	
LUNG 30,180	25%	BREAST 24,470	19%
SKIN 13,340	11%	SKIN 12,270	10%
PROSTATE 10,820	9%	LUNG 11,530	9%
BLADDER 7,800	6%	COLON 9,470	7%
COLON 7,640	6%	OVARY 5,160	4%
STOMACH 7,620	6%	STOMACH 5,130	4%
RECTUM 5,880	5%	RECTUM 4,830	4%
PANCREAS 3,330	3%	CERVIX 4,590	4%
OESOPHAGUS 2,810	2%	UTERUS 3,740	3%
LEUKAEMIA 2,649	2%	PANCREAS 3,190	2%

Source: Cancer Research Campaign

Figure 5.1: Breakdown of UK cancers.

It may be that cancer seems more prevalent nowadays because we are living longer and because we have much better diagnosis and registration systems. In the United Kingdom 70 per cent of new cases occur in people over 60 years of age; the rise in life expectancies has given cancer much more time to show itself.

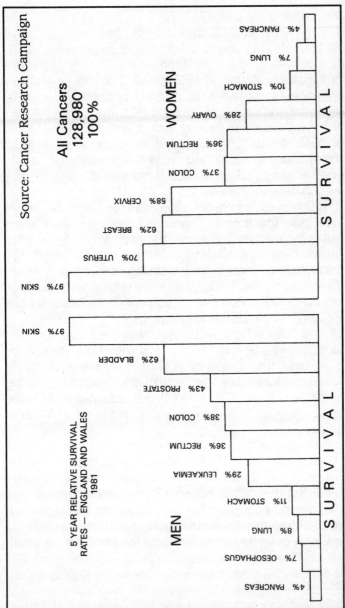

Figure 5.2: Survival rates of the ten most commonly occurring cancers in England and Wales for men and women.

Different cancers are found in varying proportions around the world. The World Health Organization has estimated that around half of all cases of cancer occur in one-fifth of the world's population, in industrial countries. The United States has similar cancer statistics to the United Kingdom: lung cancer is the biggest overall killer (particularly of men), followed by breast cancer, and cancer of the large intestine. Each year over 90,000 Americans die from lung cancer and over 44,000 from cancer of the breast. Correlations show strong links between tobacco and diet. In Australia there is a high incidence of skin cancers, including malignant melanoma: this is linked directly to over-exposure to the sun.

Vast differences in cancer rates can be seen in recent statistics put together by the Segi Institute of Cancer Epidemiology in Japan.[2] The Institute compared 36 countries from around the world using figures gathered in 1980. The report showed that there is more stomach cancer in Japan than anywhere else in the world. This is correlated with the high intake of dried, salted fish. The countries of Costa Rica and Chile follow closely in the stomach cancer table.

India and France have high rates of oral cancers, the first statistic related to the habit of chewing betel nuts, the second linked to high consumption of alcohol. Hong Kong has by far the highest rate for liver cancer, particularly in men, and also the highest rate for cancer of the oesophagus. New Zealand has the highest rate for cancer of the colon, and Hungary for cancer of the rectum.

The countries with the least incidence of all cancers were Syria, Guatemala, Saint Lucia, Thailand, Paraguay, Surinam and Panama. Why this should be the case is uncertain; it could be due to the fact that cancer registers in these countries are not very effective, or it could be that there really are less cancers. It could be that because of poor nutrition, fewer cancers take hold – it has been demonstrated that underfed mice have a much lower incidence of cancer.[3]

External Causes

Ironically, the very fact that cancer is so widespread and so varied provides important implications in the search for its causes. Through examining the figures, statisticians can see correlations between cancer risk and external factors. Such conclusions cannot be considered proof that a certain factor is without doubt a cause, but it can prompt further work on the common factors that continue to crop up in the lifestyles of people with cancer.

The concept that cancer could have external causes was first suggested by Dr Percival Pott in 1775. He noticed that cancer of the scrotum was common in men who had worked as chimney sweeps during their boyhood. In those days, small boys were made to climb up tall chimneys to clean them, and so they were regularly covered in soot; Dr Pott suggested that soot could be the cause of the cancer. It wasn't until 100 years later that a chemical in soot was found to be carcinogenic.

Some correlations have been proved: for example asbestos can definitely cause cancer, as can cigarettes and high doses of radiation. Other correlations are still being explored and take longer to prove: for example a higher intake of fresh fruit and vegetables seems to point to a lower risk of lung cancer. A similar scenario has been suggested for breast cancer, which could be linked to over-consumption of dietary fat, particularly saturated animal fat.

No one has yet been able to prove that either of the last two examples are the whole cause – the whole story – but it could be that – combined with other factors, such as genetic susceptibility inherited from blood relatives, unusual hormonal activity, and individual health – an external factor such as diet is able to tip the balance and increase the likelihood of a cancer developing.

In scientific terms there is relatively little concrete research to thoroughly convince people to change their lifestyles. Yet, in the words of a television soap detective, it's the best hunch we've got. It is believed by many scientists – although not substantiated – that cancer can be triggered and promoted by external causes. No one likes to change the habits of a lifetime, but if change can offer better protection from the frightening potential of cancer then it is surely worth considering.

Agent or circumstances	Exposure	
	Occupational	Medical
Aflatoxin		
Alcoholic drinks		
Alkylating agents:		
Cyclophosphamide		+
Melphalan		+
Aromatic amines:		
4-Aminodiphenyl	+	
Benzidine	+	
2-Naphthylamine	+	
Arsenic	+	+
Asbestos	+	
Benzene	+	
Bis(chloromethyl) ether	+	
Bisulphan		+
Cadmium	+	
Chewing (betel, tobacco, lime)		
Chromium	+	
Chlornaphazine		+
Furniture manufacture (hardwood)	+	
Immunosuppressive drugs		+
Ionizing radiations	+	+
Isopropyl alcohol manufacture	+	
Leather goods manufacture	+	
Mustard gas	+	
Nickel	+	
Oestrogens:		
Unopposed		+
Transplacental (DES)		+
Overnutrition (causing obesity)		
Phenacetin		+
Polycyclic hydrocarbons	+	+
Reproductive history:		
Late age at 1st pregnancy		
Zero or low parity		
Parasites:		
Schistosoma haematobium		
Chlonorchis sinensis		
Sexual promiscuity		
Steroids:		
Anabolic (oxymetholone)		+
Contraceptives		+
Tobacco smoking		
UV light	+	
Vinyl chloride	+	
Virus (hepatitis B)		

Source: The Causes of Cancer

Figure 5.3: Established human carcinogenic agents and circumstances.

Social	Site of cancer
+	Liver
+	Mouth, pharynx, larynx, oesophagus, liver
	Bladder
	Marrow
	Bladder
	Bladder
	Bladder
	Skin, lung
	Lung, pleura, peritoneum
	Marrow
	Lung
	Marrow
	Prostate
+	Mouth
	Lung
	Bladder
	Nasal sinuses
	Reticuloendothelial system
	Marrow and probably all other sites
	Nasal sinuses
	Nasal sinuses
	Larynx, lung
	Nasal sinuses, lung
	Endometrium
	Vagina
+	Endometrium, gall bladder
	Kidney (pelvis)
	Skin, scrotum, lung
+	Breast
+	Ovary
+	Bladder
+	Liver (cholangioma)
+	Cervix uteri
	Liver
	Liver (hamartoma)
+	Mouth, pharynx, larynx, lung, oesophagus, bladder
+	Skin, lip
	Liver (angiosarcoma)
+	Liver (hepatoma)

What Proof is There?

Examining the trends of cancer in migratory groups gives further credence to the hypothesis that lifestyle does affect cancer rates. The eminent British epidemiologists (health statisticians) Richard Doll and Richard Peto did so in their book *The Causes of Cancer.*[4]

Doll and Peto found that black Americans suffer from similar cancers as white Americans, although genetically they are of West African origin. They concluded that new factors peculiar to the American way of life must have had an influence on the types of cancer developed. If cancer was simply linked to the genetic factors of race and descent, the black Americans would have reflected the cancer rates found in West Africa.

Doll and Peto looked at figures, put together by the International Agency for Research into Cancer, which showed that cancers common in Ibadan, Nigeria, such as liver and lymphosarcoma (cancer of the lymphatic system) were much rarer in the American population of black people descended from Ibadan. The American Nigerians had much higher levels of lung and breast cancer, like their Caucasian counterparts.

The Causes of Cancer goes on to compare the cancer rates of the Japanese population with people of Japanese extraction living in Hawaii. For every type of cancer, except lung, the incidence of cancer in Hawaiian Japanese resembled that of their Caucasian neighbours. Cancers of the prostate, breast, colon and rectum were high in Hawaii, but low in Japan. Strikingly the rates of stomach cancer in Japan were four times higher than the rates shown by the Hawaiian Japanese.

Other examples cited in the book are Indians who moved to Fiji and South Africa who had a much lower risk of oral cancer, and white Britons who went to Fiji and increased their risk of skin cancer. The lower risk suffered by the Indians is thought to be because they no longer chewed carcinogenic betel nuts. The Britons are likely to have been much fairer-skinned than the native Fijians, increasing their risk of skin cancer from over-exposure to the sun.

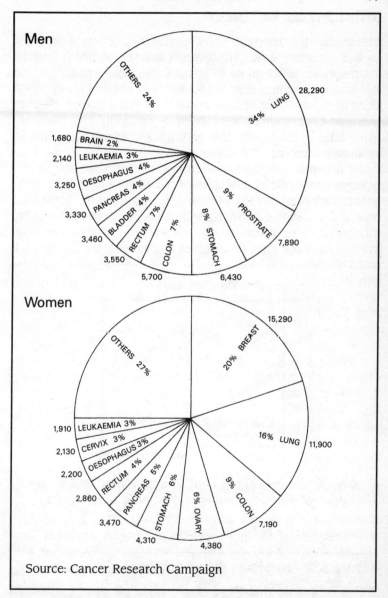

Source: Cancer Research Campaign

Figure 5.4: Breakdown of deaths in UK through cancer.

Tobacco and Cancer

The relationship between smoking and lung cancer is the most well-documented and causative yet to be established. Current estimates suggest that up to 30 per cent of cancers are caused by smoking. In the United Kingdom lung cancer accounts for a third of male cancer deaths, and it is reported that nine out of ten lung cancer cases are caused by smoking. This does not even take into account the contribution smoking makes to respiratory and heart disease.

In the United Kingdom smoking became popular in 1910 and a marked increase in cancer was noticed in 1930. In the United States the large-scale use of cigarettes began during the Second World War, leading to increased levels of cancer now. Early cigarettes were much more vicious than the modern-day variety, having higher tar content and no filters.

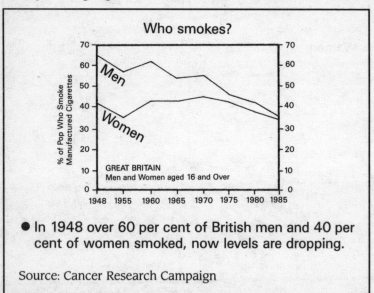

● In 1948 over 60 per cent of British men and 40 per cent of women smoked, now levels are dropping.

Source: Cancer Research Campaign

Figure 5.5: Analysis of British smokers.

It has been said that there is no single measure that would decrease deaths from cancer as much as a reduction in smoking. In late-middle-aged smokers the incidence of lung cancer is ten times that of non-smokers, and it is also thought that smoking effects cancers of the mouth, pharynx, larynx, oesophagus, bladder and possibly pancreas and kidney. Evidence suggests that smoking cigarettes doubles the chance of developing cancer of the bladder and pancreas; this is possibly due to components of cigarette smoke being absorbed into the bloodstream and then being removed through urine. Interestingly, in the United States, the rates for younger generations of smokers who have been brought up on low-tar cigarettes are slightly lower.

According to ASH, the anti-smoking campaign, lung cancer in the UK caused by smoking claims 40,000 lives every year. Recent research has suggested that passive smoking causes 300 deaths every year. One cigarette contains 30,000 different chemical compounds, including nicotine, tar, benzene, ammonia, hydrogen cyanide and formaldehyde. Of these substances 60 are known carcinogens. Cigarette smoke is therefore a potent mixture of interacting chemicals which can both initiate and promote cancer.

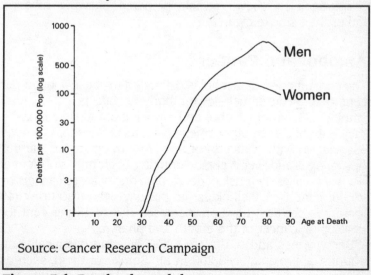

Source: Cancer Research Campaign

Figure 5.6: Deaths through lung cancer.

In the United Kingdom, smokers are now in the minority, with one in three people smoking. However, the habit is not dying out – one-fifth of 15-year-olds smoke on a regular basis, particularly girls. The temptations are very strong: each year the tobacco industry spends £113 million on advertising in the print media alone – compare this to the £5 million spent on smoking prevention programmes.

The good news is that even those who smoke heavily can increase their potential lifespan by between 10 and 15 years if they give up the habit. If they give up before fully developing cancer they avoid nearly all risk of dying from the effects of tobacco.

The links between cancer and tobacco given so much publicity in Western countries have forced companies to seek out new markets for their products. Third World countries, particularly in Africa, have become a focus of attention for cigarette marketing. In the next 20 to 30 years we may well see alarming rises in the cases of lung cancer in these parts of the world. America is experiencing a new phenomenon which may also affect statistics in several decades' time: children are being encouraged to chew specially-prepared chewing tobacco, rather than smoke cigarettes.

Alcohol and Cancer

The consumption of alcohol is estimated to cause about 3 per cent of cancers, much lower than the effects of cigarette smoking. However, alcohol and smoking are closely linked – they enhance each other's negative effects. Alcohol has been associated with cancers of the mouth, pharynx, larynx, oesophagus and liver. A person drinking 10 grammes of alcohol a day increases their risk of developing one of these cancers by 20 per cent. Heavy smokers (40 per day) who also drink (40 grammes per day) have an increased risk of 15 per cent for developing cancer of the mouth and pharynx.[5]

Beers, wines and spirits are full of different chemical compounds, approximately 1,200 in all. Somke of them, such as urethane and N-nitroso compounds, are known carcinogens.

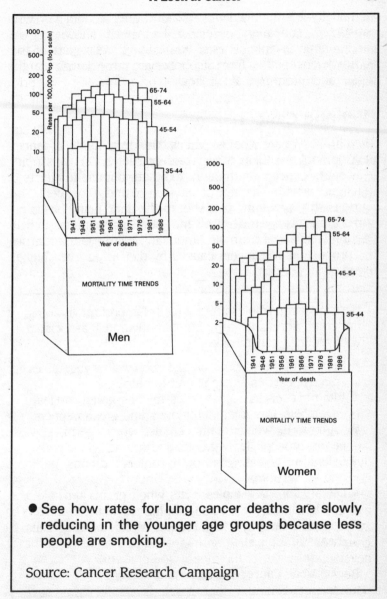

- See how rates for lung cancer deaths are slowly reducing in the younger age groups because less people are smoking.

Source: Cancer Research Campaign

Figure 5.7: Lung cancer in the UK.

Acetaldehyde is the main waste product after alcohol has been consumed and metabolized. It has been shown to be carcinogenic in animal tests. White blood cells (part of the body's defence) taken from alcoholics are more damaged than those taken from non-alcoholics.

Diet and Cancer

The phrase 'We are what we eat' is thought to apply to cancer development as well as other health problems. On average, 35 per cent of cancers are thought to be attributable to diet, and that figure is within a range of between 10 and 70 per cent. The figure is still something of a shot in the dark, being based on correlations discovered by Doll and Peto. Some experts, such as Dr John Weisburger from the American Health Foundation, put the proportion of cancers caused by diet at an even higher figure of 50 per cent.

Here are some wholesome sources of important vitamins, minerals, fibre and complex carbohydrates associated with reduced cancer risk:

- Beta-carotene: dark green and deep yellow vegetables, spinach, carrots, broccoli and tomatoes.
- Vitamin C: citrus fruits, berries, melons, green and leafy vegetables, tomatoes, cauliflower and green peppers.
- Vitamin E: whole grain cereals, wheat germ, soya beans, broccoli, leafy greens and spinach.
- Selenium: wheat germ, bran, tunafish, onions, garlic and mushrooms.
- Dietary fibre: vegetables, fruits, whole grains and baked goods containing whole grain flours.
- Complex carbohydrates: breads, cereals and legumes (beans and peas).

Source: World Cancer Research Fund

Most scientists tend to opt for the 35 per cent figure, which in itself numbers one-third of all cancer cases. The race is now on to substantiate the suggestions, in the words of Dr Weisburger it is 'an area of active current research'. Diet has been notably linked with cancers of the breast, bowel, pancreas, and stomach (the digestive system) and could have a protective effect over cancers of the lung, large bowel, oesophagus and stomach.

Doll and Peto suggested five reasons how diet could be an important factor in the cancer story:

1. By ingesting carcinogens directly from food.
2. By helping the formation of other carcinogens in the body.
3. By affecting the transport or activation of carcinogens.
4. By 'promoting' cancer in cells that have already been initiated.
5. By overeating.

There are several kinds of studies that can be done to find out the importance of diet. The first type is a case-control, where people diagnosed with cancer are interviewed about their dietary habits and compared with those who do not have cancer.

The second type is a prospective study, where a large number of people have their diets analysed and are then followed for several years to see who develops what. These studies are difficult to organize, but give a clearer idea of what sort of foods could be increasing or decreasing cancer risk. Lastly, there are intervention studies, these give direct information about whether something has an effect or not. In an intervention trial, a diet is supplemented with a particular product to see whether those being given it gain any benefit. Intervention trials require a lot of people (often around 20,000) to gain reliable statistical evidence; because of this they also need a lot of funding. These trials are the last in a long list of experiments to gauge the role of a given substance.

To date, associations linking diet with the progression of cancer have been made with fat, cholesterol, animal protein, salt, N-nitroso compounds and over-eating. Let us look at the major arguments for and against each.

Fat

The current interest in fat and breast cancer has been generated because different European countries vary so greatly in breast cancer rates. The campaigning group Europe Against Cancer is supporting several studies at the moment. The United Kingdom has the highest rate of breast cancer in the world, and the rates for northern Europe in general are six times higher than for southern Europe.

Fat is thought to be involved in the promotion of cancer, rather than in the initiation. At the moment fat makes up around 40 per cent of total energy in the British diet. Tests on animals have shown that the number of tumours in breast, bowel, pancreas and prostate cancer increase when the animals are fed a high-fat diet,[6] and that fibre can have a protective effect against fat.[7,8]

Epidemiological surveys have observed a strong link between fat and certain cancers in humans.[9,10] However, the debate continues, as tests on humans have not proved this hypothesis. The favourite theory is that, in breast cancer, fat increases levels of circulating oestrogens (female hormones), which are important promoters of breast cancer; and, in bowel cancer, fats cause an increased level of faecal bile acids, which in turn promote cancer.

Despite a lack of definitive proof, the United States National Research Council has judged that the evidence is sufficient to recommend a reduction in dietary saturated and unsaturated fats.

Cholesterol

High dietary cholesterol levels have been linked with large bowel cancer in animal studies. The rates of bowel cancer in humans are highest in countries where cholesterol intake is high. In a study of 92,000 Swedes, those with levels in excess of 6.5 micromoles of cholesterol per litre of blood had a 60 per cent greater risk of developing large bowel cancer. However, other studies have shown contrasting results, and the proposition remains inconclusive.

Meat and Animal Protein

Correlations drawn from statistics also show an increased cancer risk from consumption of meat and animal protein. It is thought that high-protein diets lead to greater levels of ammonia in the large bowel, and that ammonia is carcinogenic. Studies of Seventh Day Adventists, who are vegetarian, show that they have a lesser incidence of large bowel cancer.[11] But just to put a spanner in the works, Mormons, who are not vegetarian, also have lower levels.[12] As with all the other areas so far discussed, more solid evidence is needed.

Salt

It has been suggested that in many countries the halving of death rates from stomach cancer is due to better methods of food preservation and preparation. We no longer rely so much on salt and curing processes to preserve our food. In Japan, cancer of the stomach is more common than any other type, and there is a strong correlation between this and the amount of dried, salted fish consumed.

A study recently completed by Dr Brian Henderson, of the University of Southern California, showed that Hong Kong Chinese who had consistently eaten Cantonese-style salted fish from infancy upwards had a risk of contracting nasopharyngeal cancer over seven times greater than those who did not eat the fish.

Any risk from salt may be further compounded by a lack of fresh fruit and vegetables, which appear to have a protective effect. Some scientists believe this factor could be much more important than salt.

N-Nitroso Compounds

These chemical compounds are some of the most powerful carcinogens to be tested in the laboratory. They are formed from the ingestion of nitrates or nitrites in the stomach or bladder. Nitrite can be used as a preservative or colour and flavour enhancer in foods, and nitrates can be absorbed through food and water.

N-nitroso compounds have been linked to stomach and

bowel cancer, but it appears from research carried out at the Louisiana State University Medical School by Dr Pelayo Correa, that those whose main nitrate source was from fruits and vegetables had a lower risk of pre-cancerous changes (mutations of the cells). This area still needs a lot more research.

Over-Eating

Last but not least, obesity from over-eating is thought to add to the risk of developing cancer. In animal studies a 20 per cent reduction in food intake suppresses tumour formation by 60 per cent if foodstuffs are natural, and 40 per cent if they are synthetic.[13]

In relation to humans, a study by the American Cancer Society has shown that breast and endometrial (uterus) cancer were increased in women who were 40 per cent above average weight. An increase in these cancers has also been observed in post-menopausal women, which is thought to be linked to the production of certain hormones.

Fibre

The consumption of fibre has for some time been associated with a lower incidence of large-bowel cancer. Fibre is found in fruits, vegetables, legumes and wholegrain foods. The suggestion was first made after research twenty years ago revealed that rural Africans ate more fibre than Europeans, and suffered far fewer bowel cancers.

Since that time, this theory about rural Africans has been disproved, but interest in fibre still continues. Work looking at diet in the United Kingdom during the Second World War has found that cancers of the breast and colon decreased as the intake of sugar, meat and fat went down. At the same time intake of fibre via cereals and vegetables increased.[14]

It is suggested that if fibre does have a protective effect it is because it speeds up the exit of waste food materials from the bowel – allowing carcinogenic substances less time to interact. Professor John Marks of Girton College, Cambridge, has said that fibre could reduce the amount of carcinogenic steroids derived from the bile acids in the small intestine. Fibre also increases the bulk of a stool, possibly diluting any carcinogenic content.

The UK Department of Health recently stated:

> Case-control studies of fibre and large-bowel cancer have not yielded a consistent argument either for or against a protective effect . . . The majority of studies of controls compared with cases since 1975 have shown a reduction in risk, but usually as a result of increased vegetable consumption, rather than cereal fibre.[15]

One study compared Finnish and Danish groups with similar fat intakes. Cancer of the colon was far lower in the rural Finnish group than in the Danes of Copenhagen. The Finns had a high-fibre diet, containing lots of rye bread, whereas the Danes had very low fibre intakes.[16]

The US National Research Council's Committee on Diet, Nutrition and Cancer reviewed the findings of a study which said that a lower incidence of colon cancer was linked with the pentose part of fibre. The study claimed that this effect depended upon the type of fibre consumed and the chemical carcinogen involved.[17] In 1982 the Research Council recommended that further studies should look at types of fibre rather than fibre as a whole. Studies in Europe and the United States continue to look for an answer.

Vitamin C and E

Low levels of vitamins C and E in the blood have been linked with cancers of the oesophagus, larynx, stomach and oral cavity. These vitamins are usually obtained through the diet from citrus fruits, vegetables, vegetable oils, whole grains, liver and beans.

Although there is still a great need for further research into their mechanisms, it is believed that vitamins C and E may have a preventive effect on cancer because they are powerful antioxidants (see Chapter 8), and may prevent the initial damage to DNA and/or the trigger damage that leads to cancer.

Antioxidant vitamins can have an effect on the formation of N-nitroso compounds in the stomach and are therefore linked with cancer of the digestive tract. Studies in northern Iran have shown that diets low in fruits and vegetables may contribute to cancer of the oesophagus.[18,19] Similar deficiencies reported in some Chinese provinces may also contribute to the higher incidence of this type of cancer.[20] Another study, using rats, has shown that oral vitamin C blocks the tumour formation after the implantation of a known carcinogen.[21]

Other indications are that the two vitamins could prevent the formation of a mutagenenic (DNA damaging) substance called fecapentane which occurs in the bowel. Whether this has any effect on the development of bowel polyps is being investigated. A trial discussed briefly in the UK Department of Health's booklet *Diet and Cancer* showed that the recurrence of colorectal polyps was reduced by 20 per cent in patients given 400 mg each of vitamins C and E daily.[22]

Selenium

Selenium is a trace mineral found naturally in very small amounts in the body. It is absorbed from foods such as animal organs, grains and seafoods. Numerous research studies on animals have shown that selenium has a very definite anti-tumour effect. They suggest a protective effect on cancers of the lung, breast, bowel and prostate.

Statistical correlations have been found in the north-eastern United States between industrialization, high intake of dietary fat, and low soil selenium (as a mineral, it is found in the soil). However one study has shown that selenium levels in the body decline as the cancer progresses, suggesting that a lowering of selenium is possibly a result of cancer.[23] Further studies of selenium are continuing in China, Finland and the United States.

Vitamin A and Beta-Carotene

Vitamin A and beta-carotene have been major subjects of examination by the medical and scientific professions for over 15 years. The American National Cancer Institute, which established its chemoprevention research programme in 1980, did a lot of its initial work on vitamin A and beta-carotene. Now the Institute is involved in funding 12 more case-control and intervention studies to look at the possibilities of vitamin A and beta-carotene.

In recent years, the spotlight has been on beta-carotene, which has shown promising links in lowering the risk of cancers of the lung, stomach, mouth and possibly cervix and bladder. However, scientists have not yet been able to rule out the effects of vitamin A on cancer; it is known to have an integral role in the control of cell proliferation, whereas beta-carotene is an antioxidant and powerful singlet oxygen quencher (see Chapter 8), and may be involved in preventing damage to DNA. Beta-carotene's role in cancer prevention will be discussed further in Chapter 6.

Can We Fight Cancer?

The answer is a resounding 'yes'. Research so far has shown that there are many possibilities that could help to prevent cancer. Smoking habits can be changed if people are made aware of the risks; eating a diet full of fruit and vegetables, fibre and unrefined food products, with occasional animal protein and fat, is a good way to ensure that your body is in optimum health.

The links so far observed between diet and cancer are so strong that scientific proof must eventually be forthcoming. In both Europe and the United States governments have begun to re-educate people about diet. The newly launched organization, Europe Against Cancer, is aiming to reduce European cancer rates by 15 per cent by the end of the century. It is a big goal, but one the organization thinks it can meet. Avoiding external causes will undoubtedly play a big part.

Europe Against Cancer's 'Code for Living' is being publicized in every country, in order to raise awareness about the importance of diet and lifestyle in the development of cancer. The code includes such advice as don't smoke, drink moderately, avoid excessive exposure to the sun, and eat plenty of fresh fruit and vegetables.

Similar information is being given out in the United States by the National Cancer Institute. Its booklet, *Diet, Nutrition & Cancer Prevention: The Good News*, recommends avoiding fatty foods, sugar and salt, and increasing consumption of foods rich in starch and fibre, such as fruit, vegetables and cereals.

World Cancer Research Fund Dietary Guidelines to Lower Cancer Risk

1. To reduce the intake of total dietary fat from the current average of approximately 42% to a level of 30% of total calories and reduce the intake of saturated fat to less than 10% of total calories.
2. Increase the consumption of fruits, vegetables and whole grain cereals.
3. Consume salt-cured, salt-pickled and smoked foods only in moderation.
4. Drink alcohol in moderation, if at all.

Source: World Cancer Research Fund

Professor Pryor of Louisiana State University said at a recent conference on the subject:

> If micronutrients can modify the disease process we are looking at a bright new frontier, preventing horrible, life-shortening diseases with what are really quite simple means.[24]

Cancer is an extremely complicated disease, and cannot be regarded as something to be treated with a pill or a potion. The causes are manifold and individual, but there *is* hope and progression in our understanding of the disease. The future looks brighter than it has for some time.

Notes

1. Doll, R. *et al., The Causes of Cancer*, Oxford Medical Publications, Oxford, 1981.

2. Hattori, H. *et al.*, *Age-adjusted Death Rates for Cancer for Selected Sites in 36 Countries in 1980*, Segi Institute of Cancer Epidemiology, Japan, September, 1987.
3. Willet, W.C., 'Implications of total energy intake for epidemiologic studies of breast and bowel cancer', *American Journal of Clinical Nutrition*, 1987, 45, pp. 354–60.
4. See 1.
5. *Monographs on the Evaluation of Carcinogenic Risk to Humans: Alcohol Drinking*, International Agency for Research on Cancer, Lyon, 44, 1987.
6. Palmer, S. *et al.*, 'Diet, nutrition and cancer 1: interim dietary guidelines', *Journal of the National Cancer Institute*, 1983, pp. 1151–70.
7. Trudel, J.L. *et al.*, 'The fat/fibre antagonism in experimental colon carcinogenesis', *Surgery*, 94(4), 1983, pp. 691–6.
8. Reddy, B.S. *et al.*, 'Effect of dietary corn bran and autohydrolyzed lignen on 3,2-dimenthyl-4-aminobiphenyl-induced intestinal carcinogenesis in male F344 rats', *Journal of the National Cancer Institute*, 71(2), 1983, pp. 419–23.
9. See 5.
10. Waterhouse, J. *et al.*, *Cancer Incidence in Five Continents*, vol. 3, International Agency for Research on Cancer, Lyon, 15, 1976.
11. Phillips, R.L., 'Role of lifestyle and dietary habits in risk of cancer among Seventh Day Adventists', *Cancer Research*, 1975, 35, pp. 3515–22.
12. Lyon, J.L. *et al.*, 'Cancer incidence in Mormons and non-Mormons in Utah during 1967–75', *Journal of the National Cancer Institute*, 1980a, 65, pp. 1055–61.
13. Willet, W.C., 'Implications of total energy intake for epidemiologic studies of breast and bowel cancer', *American Journal of Nutrition*, 45, 1987, pp. 354–60.
14. Ingram, D.M., 'Trends in diet and breast cancer mortality in England and Wales 1928–1977', *Nutrition and Cancer*, 1981, 3(2), pp. 75–80.
15. *Diet and Cancer*, Department of Health, 1989.
16. MacLennan, R. *et al.*, 'Diet, transit time, stool weight, and colon cancer in two Scandivanian populations', *American*

Journal of Clinical Nutrition, 31, 1978, pp. S239–42.

17. Bingham, S. *et al.*, 'Dietary fibre and regional large-bowel cancer mortality in Britain', *British Journal of Cancer*, 40, 1979, pp. 456–63.

18. Joint Iran-International Agency for Research on Cancer Study Group, Oesophageal cancer studies in the Caspian littoral of Iran: results of population studies – a podrome', *Journal of the National Cancer Institute*, 59, 1977, pp. 1127–138.

19. Cook-Mozaffari, P.J. *et al.*, 'Oesophageal cancer studies in the Caspian littoral of Iran: results of a case control study', *British Journal of Cancer*, 39, 1979, pp. 293–309.

20. Yang, C.S. *et al.*, New Jersey medical School, Newark NJ, Cancer Institute of Chinese Academy of Medical Sciences, Beijing, and NCI, Bethesda, Md, oral presentation at *Vitamin A and Cancer Prevention Conference*, NIH, Bethesda, Md, February 28–29, 1984.

21. Pipkin, G.E. *et al.*, 'Inhibitory effect of L-ascorbate on tumour formation in urinary bladders implanted with 3-hydroxynathranilic acid', *Proceedings of the Society of Experimental Biology*, 131, 1969, pp. 522–24.

22. Willett, W.C. *et al.*, 'Relation of serum vitamins C and E to the risk of cancer', *New England Journal of Medicine*, 310, 1984, pp. 430–34.

23. Virtamo, J. *et al.*, 'Serum selenium and the risk of cancer', *Cancer*, 60, 1987, pp. 145–48.

24. Antioxidant Vitamins and beta-carotene in disease prevention, conference, London, September 1989. Hosted by Roche.

Chapter 6

Beta-Carotene and Cancer Prevention

The prevention, rather than the cure, of cancer is now a central aim of doctors and scientists involved in the field of treatment and research. For many years now, a search has been conducted, often quietly, for substances that will prevent cancer from ever taking hold.

The term used by doctors for this process is 'chemo-prevention', described as an attempt 'to arrest or reverse pre-malignant cells during their progression to invasive malignancy'.[1] This means stopping the mutant cells mentioned in the last chapter from turning into anything more serious. The theory is that cancer can be brought to a halt by intervening with both natural and synthetic substances – for example micronutrients such as vitamins and minerals.

The development of a chemopreventive substance goes through several stages, including cell culture work, tests on animals (usually mice and rats) and finally intervention trials on human beings. The National Cancer Institute (NCI) of the United States is currently funding 18 intervention trials to see whether or not specific substances can stop cancer. For each chosen substance there will already be a wealth of positive background information available, and the doctors organizing the trial will be pretty confident of good results.

Out of the 18 trials sponsored by the NCI, seven of them involve beta-carotene and four of them vitamin A (known to scientists as retinol). The beta-carotene trials cover cancer of the lung, mouth, colon, skin, and one organized by Harvard Medical School's Professor Charles Hennekens will look at all sites; vitamin A is being dispensed in relation to lung and mouth cancers.[2]

For a single nutrient to feature in just under half the influential NCI intervention trials is impressive progress, but it is only the result of many years of painstaking data collection about beta-carotene (see Chapter 7 for main studies). Statistical studies have shown a clear link between dietary intake of fruits and vegetables and a lower risk of certain cancers; there is strong evidence that the active ingredient could be beta-carotene. Research is continuing to try and establish this link as a solid fact, and also to explore further capabilities of carotenoids in general.

Statistical evidence gleaned from the study of human patterns of disease shows the strongest links between beta-carotene and cancer of the lung. There is a weaker association with cancer of the stomach. Together with vitamin A, beta-carotene has also shown preventive effects against oral leukoplakia, a pre-malignant state in oral cancer. Tests on mice, rats and hamsters have shown that beta-carotene can regress and protect against cancers of the skin, breast, colon and bladder.[3]

Most of these cancers are of the epithelial tissues, the mucous inner linings of the body, such as the digestive and respiratory tracts. The animal research has not yet been repeated in humans, but the results are strong enough to provoke further research in these areas. Interestingly, vitamin A plays a vital role in the health of these mucous linings. Once beta-carotene has been digested it concentrates in the adipose layer of tissues, the fatty parts; this could perhaps explain in part why it is protective in animal models of skin and breast cancer.

How the Research Began

Research into this corner of the micronutrient field began seventy years ago, when a scientist named Mori noticed that a deficiency of vitamin A led to changes in the mucous lining of the respiratory tract.[4] His discovery prompted a mini-flurry of interest in other scientific laboratories, and in 1925, three years after Mori had submitted his research paper for publication, Doctors Wolbach and Howe made the same observations, but this time in the mucous lining of the stomach and bladder.[5]

In 1926, Fujimake made a giant leap in association by showing that rats fed a vitamin A-deficient diet would develop stomach tumours, made even worse when carcinogens were administered.[6]

It wasn't until the 1930s that the concept of prevention by administration of beta-carotene was illustrated. Scientists found that if vitamin A-deficient rats were fed beta-carotene, infections of the ear, bladder, kidney and gut were all prevented.[7] Another study, this time looking at dietary supplementation in human beings, concluded that severe earache in young children was helped following an increase in the amount of carotene-rich foods eaten.[8]

Since that time, studies on vitamin A, beta-carotene and a few other carotenoids like canthaxanthin, lutein and lycopene have come thick and fast. They have brought with them an endless source of debate, hope and frustration. However, the shift in emphasis towards beta-carotene came with the publication in 1981 of an influential report by Richard Doll and Richard Peto, entitled *Can Dietary Beta-Carotene Materially Reduce Human Cancer Rates?*[9] It reviewed the evidence available and sparked off a whole new burst of enthusiasm, hence all the NCI studies.

Ten years on, Richard Peto remains uncompromisingly sceptical of the claims that beta-carotene could have a protective effect against cancer, even though he and his colleagues originally gave it such a positive write-up. He represents one end of the scientific spectrum which refuses to believe anything until there is irresistible proof. While Peto plays the whole issue down, others are prepared to stick their necks out and speak more positively in beta-carotene's favour.

Dr Regina Ziegler of the NCI was prepared to do so at a recent international conference on beta-carotene and antioxidants where she said:

When the reduced risk of lung cancer observed with vegetable and fruit and carotenoid intake in dietary studies is combined with the reduced risk of lung cancer observed with low levels of beta-carotene in serum and plasma [blood] studies, the simplest, though not the only explanation, is that beta-carotene is protective.[10]

There are always two sides to the coin.

The Story Behind Vitamin A

For a long time, the main thrust of research was aimed at finding a mechanism by which vitamin A could work. It was thought that beta-carotene had no other biological function except as a precursor of vitamin A. Scientists firmly believed that if anything was the answer this was it. Certain cancers appeared to be preventible through the action of vitamin A on the body's metabolism.

As an assumption, it was a reasonable one to make, and one that has not yet been dismissed. Without vitamin A the human body does develop deficiency symptoms; it is essential for healthy skin and the health of the inner mucous membranes which line the respiratory tract, the digestive system, the colon and the bladder. The epithelial tissues are designed to be waterproof, stretchy and protective.

It is well known that vitamin A has a small but important role to play in controlling cell differentiation – the process whereby cells are equipped for various functions. The logical progression therefore, is that vitamin A could stop a mutant cell from turning cancerous.

In animal and cell culture tests, vitamin A has been linked with cancers of the respiratory system, breast and bladder.[11] In humans it has been most commonly associated with lung and mouth cancer. Out of five current NCI intervention trials concentrating on lung cancer, three are including a comparison between vitamin A and beta-carotene. This shows that scientists want to see if either of the two nutrients is more effective. The results could show that they both work well, but in different ways.

Dr David Thurnham, a senior scientist at the Dunn Nutrition

Centre in Cambridge, has another interesting theory about the role of vitamin A in cancer prevention. He believes that vitamin A levels in tissue could act as an early warning system that the body is in a state of flux before a disease takes hold.

In a review concerning malaria, submitted to the *Transactions of the Royal Society of Tropical Medicine*, Dr Thurnham stated that vitamin A was an 'acute phase reactant'. In populations with malaria, he found that although patients shouldn't have been deficient in vitamin A, they had all suffered similar drops in levels in the blood.[12]

When a person enters a state of stress, the veins and arteries become more permeable, allowing large protein complexes to float away from the blood stream and into the tissues. Vitamin A is bound to a large protein complex, and therefore would be a part of this process.

Dr Thurnham believes that low levels of vitamin A in the blood could simply be predictive of a disease state in the body, rather than a possible cause. Although he has no firm evidence yet, Dr Thurnham intends to concentrate on analysing blood samples, to see whether vitamin A levels go down when the body is ill, and up when it is better.

The Story Behind Beta-Carotene

The interest in vitamin A and cancer prevention is still strong, but the emphasis has shifted to beta-carotene, mainly because there is such a strong correlation between high intake of foods containing beta-carotene (fruits and vegetables) and lower risks of certain cancers, particularly lung and stomach. Worldwide, 60 dietary studies looking into beta-carotene have been completed. For foods simply rich in pure vitamin A (fish liver oil, eggs, dairy products) the association is not found. Beta-carotene, in its own right, is now the focus of attention.

No one has yet come up with enough substantial evidence to prove exactly why beta-carotene should have a protective effect against some cancers, but experiments have shown that beta-carotene acts as an antioxidant which scavenges free radicals, and is also an efficient quencher of singlet oxygen (see

Vegetable or fruit	Carotenoid or carotenoid class (mg of carotenoid/100 g of edible food)				
	Lutein	Epoxy carotenoids	Alpha carotene	Beta carotene	Lycopene
Broccoli, raw	2.06	1.70	—	0.48	—
Brussels sprouts					
Raw	1.59	2.74	—	0.53	—
Cooked	1.29	1.17	—	0.45	—
Cabbage, raw	0.31	0.50	—	0.08	—
Carrots, canned	—	—	2.80	4.76	—
Kale					
Raw	39.6	23.4	—	14.6	—
Cooked	25.6	15.2	—	12.6	—
Palm oil, red	—	—	66.9	120.5	20.0
Spinach, raw	15.9	13.8	—	6.71	—
Acorn squash					
Raw	0.38	0.11	—	0.22	—
Cooked	0.66	0.20	—	0.49	—
Strawberries	0.06	—	—	0.23	—
Sweet potatoes, canned	—	—	—	16.0	—
Tomatoes, raw	—	—	—	0.50	6.70

Source: Journal of the American National Cancer Institute

Figure 6.1: Carotenoid content of foods associated with reduction in cancer incidence rates.

Chapter 9). Free radicals and singlet oxygen are both capable of damaging DNA through chain reactions, this could produce a potentially cancerous cell.

Another group of scientists, notably the Americans Dr Adrianne Bendich and Professor Norman Krinsky, have been researching the theory that beta-carotene can also bolster up the defence cells which are capable of killing tumour cells: these are the macrophages, natural killer cells and cytotoxic T cells. Encouraging results have been gained from experiments on cell cultures and rats and mice, but scientists cannot yet tell whether the results can be repeated inside a human body.

One also has to remember that these experiments are carried out under test conditions with controlled substances and breeds of rodent which are particularly susceptible to cancer.

The environment is totally artificial, and not subject to the thousands of different reactions you would find in a human body undergoing the stresses and strains of everyday life.

Another thought-provoking suggestion, as yet unsubstantiated, from Dr Graham Burton of the National Research Council of Canada, is that beta-carotene protects against cancer because if oxidizes very quickly once inside the body. The end products of this oxidation could in turn destroy cancer cells.

In her 1989 review of the statistical evidence for beta-carotene's role in cancer prevention, Dr Regina Ziegler of the American National Cancer Institute threw another spanner in the works.[13] She reminded scientists that the role of other major carotenoids, those that will be eaten in the diet alongside beta-carotene, has not been well-researched. Dr Ziegler, who has had a long-term interest in beta-carotene, posed the question that other carotenoids commonly found in foods, such as lutein, lycopene and zeaxanthin, could help to explain the protective role. It is a suggestion more and more scientists in the field are taking seriously. The collective work on beta-carotene has brought about extra interest in other members of the carotenoid family, but for the moment all the research has been done on beta-carotene, and all the current trials involve this particular nutrient. The US National Cancer Institute has already begun to take an initial look at the effects of lutein, lycopene, beta-cryptoxanthin and alpha-carotene on cancer.

Target site organ	Target/risk group	Inhibitory agents
Lung	Chronic smokers	Folic acid Vitamin B_{12}
Lung	Men, asbestosis	Beta-carotene Retinol
Lung	Cigarette smokers	Beta-carotene Retinol
Lung	Men exposed to asbestos	Beta-carotene Retinol

Target site organ	Target/risk group	Inhibitory agents
Lung	Chronic smokers	13-cis Retinoic acid
Oral cavity	Leukoplakia	13-cis Retinoic acid
Oral cavity	Leukoplakia	Beta-carotene 13-cis Retinoic acid
Colon	Familial polyposis	Vitamin C, E, and fibre
Colon	Previous adenoma of colon	Calcium
Colon	Previous adenoma of colon	Beta-carotene, Vitamin C and E
Colon	Previous adenoma of colon	Piroxicam
Colon	Previous adenoma of colon	Fibre, calcium
Skin	Albinos in Tanzania	Beta-carotene
Skin	Previous basal bell carcinoma of skin	Beta-carotene
Skin	Actinic keratoses patients	Retinol
Skin	Previous squamous cell carcinoma or BCC of skin	Selenium
Skin	Previous BCC of skin	Retinol, 13-cis Retinoic acid
Cervix	Women, mild, moderate dysplasia	Retinyl acetate
Cervix	Women, cervical dysplasia	Folic acid
Breast	Women, previous breast cancer	4HPR
All sites	Physicians	Beta-carotene

Source: American National Cancer Institute

Figure 6.2: Chemoprevention intervention studies.

Dietary and statistical studies with human relevance have already shown great promise for beta-carotene. The current intervention trials will contradict or shore up this promise. Until these results are out, however, we can only base conclusions on work already done; the next chapter looks at all the major studies linking beta-carotene with cancer protection.

Notes

1. Sporn, M.B. *et al.*, 'Prevention of chemical carcinogenesis by vitamin A and its synthetic analogs (retinoids)', *Federation Proceedings*, 1976, 35, pp. 1332–38.
2. Malone, W.F., *Studies evaluating antioxidants and beta-carotene as chemopreventives*, Chemoprevention Branch, National Cancer Institute, Bethesda, Md, USA.
3. Santamaria, L. *et al.*, 'Cancer chemoprevention by supplemental carotenoids in animals and humans', *Preventive Medicine*, 18(5), 1989, pp. 603–23.
4. Mori, S., 'The changes in the paraocular glands which follow the administration of diets low in fat-soluble vitamin A with notes of the effects of the same diets on the salivary glands and the mucosa of the larynx and brachea', *John Hopkins Hospital Bulletin*, 1922, 33, pp. 357–59.
5. Wolbach, S.D. *et al.*, 'Tissue changes following deprivation of fat-soluble A vitamin', *Journal of Experimental Medicine*, 1925, 42, pp. 753–77.
6. Fujimake, Y., 'Formation of carcinoma in albino rats fed on deficient diets', *Journal of Cancer Research*, 1926, 10, pp. 469–77.
7. Green, H.N. *et al.*, 'Carotene and vitamin A: the anti-infective action of carotene', *British Journal of Experimental Pathology*, 11, 1930, pp. 81–9.
8. Clausen, S.W., 'Carotenemia and resistance to infection', *Transactions of the American Pediatric Society*, 1931, 43, pp. 27–30.
9. Peto, R. *et al.*, 'Can dietary beta-carotene materially reduce human cancer rates?', *Nature*, 290, 19 March 1981, pp. 201–8.

10. Antioxidant vitamins and beta-carotene in disease prevention, Conference, London, September 1989. Hosted by Roche.
11. Thurnham, D.I. and Singkamani, R., 'The acute phase response and vitamin A status in malaria', *Transactions of the Royal Society of Tropical Medicine and Hygiene*, 1991, vol. 85, in press.
12. *ibid*.
13. Ziegler, R.G., 'A review of epidemiologic evidence that carotenoids reduce the risk of cancer', *Journal of Nutrition*, 119, pp. 116–22.

Chapter 7

Beta-Carotene and Cancer Prevention: The Major Studies

Research into beta-carotene's action as a chemopreventive has been done in many parts of the world, by a great many scientists. Hundreds of minor studies have been done on cell cultures and animal models, but there have been relatively few concentrating purely on human intakes of the nutrient.

The majority of the most convincing studies show links between low levels of beta-carotene and higher risk of lung cancer. The following summaries round up the evidence in favour of beta-carotene's protective effect.

Lung Cancer

1. 'Dietary Vitamin A and Human Lung Cancer', by E. Bjelke, *International Journal of Cancer*, 15, 1975, pp. 561–65.

Bjelke's study isolated a relationship between low levels of vitamin A and lung cancer. Although he did not refine the study down to the effects of beta-carotene, it was an influential piece of work referred to in many subsequent studies.

Bjelke's study consisted of 8,278 men drawn generally from the Norwegian population, and also contained a number of men who were brothers of migrants to the United States. Sixty per cent of the men smoked to varying degrees, and were over 45 years old at the beginning of the five-year follow-up.

The study was a prospective dietary investigation, looking at what the men ate, what their smoking habits were, and where they lived. The men were surveyed twice, in 1964 and in 1967, both times with a dietary questionnaire. Eighty per cent completed the first survey, 90 per cent the second. Each food recorded in the survey was given a nutritional status and an index established for vitamin A content.

Bjelke reported that the variation in index vitamin A levels depended on intake of vegetables, particularly carrots, milk and eggs. Cases of cancer were followed up for five years following through the Norwegian Cancer Registry, which is based on all new reports of cancer. To prevent ambiguity only cases that had been classified as cancers of the bronchus and lung were included in the final results.

Between the years of 1968 and 1972, 36 cases of cancer of the lung and bronchus were diagnosed in the study population. A lower level of lung cancer was found in all groups with higher vitamin A levels. There were no notable age differences, and only four of the lung cancers occurred in the 40 per cent of men who had never smoked.

In his conclusion Bjelke wrote:

> Chance seems an unlikely explanation for the association noted . . . The present findings do suggest that vitamin A active compounds or some closely associated dietary factors may modify the expression of pulmonary carcinogens or cocarcinogens in man. In view of the difficulties of influencing smoking behaviour, the suggestion that ingested agents may be potent prophylactics against the effects of smoking should be of more than theoretical interest.

How right he was! Although there is a steady decline in smoking in the West, there are still enough people who do smoke to warrant a recommendation to increase intake of fresh fruit and vegetables. This is particularly important in the light of dietary surveys which have shown that smokers tend to have a much lower intake of fruit and vegetables than non-smokers.

Bjelke classified the active protective factor as vitamin A, but was careful to include the phrase 'or closely associated dietary factors'. This possibility was later explored by many other scientists, as the Bjelke study encouraged further examination of the phenomenon.

2. 'Dietary Vitamin A and Risk of Cancer in the Western Electric Study, by Richard B. Shekelle, *et al*, *The Lancet*, 28 November 1981.

The Western Electric study, as it is known, was a huge undertaking by Richard Shekelle and his co-researchers. Over a 19-year period, Shekelle reviewed dietary habits of 2,107 middle-aged men and recorded whether they were diagnosed with cancer. In what is regarded as a major contribution to the research done on beta-carotene, he found that lung cancer risk was associated with low levels of this nutrient, rather than to vitamin A.

In his introduction, Shekelle pinpointed an area of ambiguity that had been presented in earlier studies:

> Although some results were presented for selected groups of foods, these studies did not clearly determine whether the risk was associated with intake of preformed vitamin A (retinol), intake of provitamin A (carotene) or intake of both ... This study was undertaken to investigate the association between intake of carotene and retinol in the diet as assessed in 1959, and the risk of cancer during the following 19 years in a group of men.

This study was designed to show whether beta-carotene could have an effect independent of vitamin A. For his representative group, Shekelle went to the Western Electric Company's Hawthorne works, based in Chicago; the men he selected were involved in the manufacture of telephones.

Between 1957 and 1958 a total of 2,107 men were examined. Two nutritionists asked questions about diet at the initial examination and then again at a second examination one year later. A questionnaire was designed to determine what kinds and quantities of foods had been eaten during the previous 28 days. A one-hour interview asked participants about eating patterns during workdays and weekends, and presented them with a list of 195 types of food, to find out how often they were eaten and in what proportions. Food supplements were rarely used.

The recorded data was used to estimate the daily intake of several nutrients, including vitamin A. To classify how much of the vitamin A was taken in as beta-carotene, the analysts looked at the consumption of three food groups: vegetables, fruit and soup. The men in the study were re-examined every year until 1969.

Nine years later, Shekelle and colleagues followed up each participant, to see what had become of them. Thirty-three men had developed lung cancer; intake of the three carotene food groups for these men was comparatively low, whereas the vitamin A levels were not significantly associated. The amount of beta-carotene consumed was not related to age, but was less in those who smoked.

Men who developed lung cancer tended to have a below-average intake of dietary beta-carotene at the beginning of the study, a tendency which persisted throughout the 19 years. Shekelle concluded that levels of beta-carotene could be correlated to lung cancer risk, but not to any other type of cancer. According to the study there were no other significant differences in other nutrients between men who developed lung cancer and men who did not. Shekelle stated: 'The long period of follow-up indicates below average intake of carotene preceded the carcinoma (tumour) and was not a consequence of it.' This is a factor scientists are still trying to establish.

The Western Electric study was concluded with the following, very cautious, words:

> The consistency of epidemiological [statistical] evidence from diverse populations ... its independence from cigarette smoking, and its coherence with the evidence from animals, all suggest that a diet relatively high in beta-carotene may reduce the risk of lung cancer even among persons who have smoked cigarettes for many years.

3. 'Serum Vitamin Levels and the Risk of Cancer of Specific Sites in Men of Japanese Ancestry in Hawaii', by Abraham Nomura et al., *Cancer Research*, 45, May 1985, pp. 2369–72.

Abraham Nomura and colleagues also found a correlation between low beta-carotene levels and lung cancer, but were not quite so positive as Shekelle. The study also differed because Nomura examined blood samples using a technique called high performance liquid chromatography – the most accurate method of discovering all the variants in blood. Shekelle simply relied on dietary information and did not test his subjects' blood.

Nomura's study concentrated on a small geographical area: the island of Oahu in Hawaii. Between 1971 and 1975 they tested blood samples from 6,800 men for levels of vitamins A, E and beta-carotene. In a ten-year follow-up they decided to look for associations between cancers of the lung, stomach, colon, rectum and bladder.

When the blood samples were originally collected and tested, none of the subjects had been diagnosed with cancer. During the follow-up period, Nomura and his team scanned the hospitals of Oahu and referred to the Hawaii Tumor Registry, to discover how many of the men had since developed cancer.

From their observations, Nomura concluded that vitamins E and A could not be associated with the specific cancers mentioned. But, once again there was a strong negative association between beta-carotene blood levels and lung cancer. Beta-carotene also decreased slightly in relation to stomach and colon, but when compared to controls (people matched for age, dietary habits etc., but without cancer) it was insignificant.

Nomura concluded:

> In order to put the association of beta-carotene with lung cancer into proper perspective, it should be noted that the factor of greatest importance for lung cancer in this study population continues to be cigarette smoking . . . Furthermore, it is not known if cigarette smokers can reduce their

risk of lung cancer by increasing their intake of dietary beta-carotene.

4. 'Smoking and Other Risk Factors for Lung Cancer in Women', by Anna Wu *et al, Journal of National Cancer Institute*, vol. 74, no. 4, April 1985.

This study is interesting because it concentrates purely on women. It involved 220 women diagnosed with lung cancer: 149 had the adenocarcinoma type of cancer, another 71 squamous cell. Some smoked but some were non-smokers. A questionnaire was designed to discover smoking habits, passive smoking, lung disease and vitamin A intake.

The section on vitamin A intake included specific questions on the frequency of consumption of 21 vegetables and fruits, all high in beta-carotene. Wu and colleagues observed a significant decrease in risk for both types of cancer with a high intake of these kinds of foods. This result echoes those of trials which have looked specifically at men.

5. 'Serum Beta-Carotene, Vitamins A and E, Selenium, and the Risk of Lung Cancer, by Marilyn S. Menkes *et al, The New England Journal of Medicine*, 315, pp. 1250–54.

In this study, often known as the Washington County study, Marilyn Menkes and her team found a strong correlation between low levels of beta-carotene in the blood and risk of lung cancer, but managed to whittle down the results even further by isolating the type of lung cancer with which it was most strongly associated. In 1974 a large blood survey took place in Washington County, Maryland. It numbered 25,802 people ranging from 25 to 64 years old. Out of this huge pool of people, 99 were subsequently diagnosed with lung cancer between 1975 and 1983. Menkes matched up these 99 people to 196 controls (who had not got cancer, but were of similar age, sex, race, smoking habits and month of blood collection), and then had all their blood samples analysed, using high performance liquid chromatography.

Menkes found that there was no association between low

vitamin A levels and lung cancer, but that the risk of lung cancer increased with decreasing levels of beta-carotene and vitamin E. There was a particularly strong correlation between one type of lung cancer – squamous cell – and low beta-carotene levels.

Menkes realized that the significantly lower levels of vitamin E and beta-carotene in the blood samples of those diagnosed with cancer could have been a result of pre-malignant changes caused by the cancer. However, she dismissed this concern, because there were no falling or rising trends over time when cases were tested at three-year intervals and compared to their controls.

In her summary, Menkes questioned whether the lessening of lung cancer risk through beta-carotene could be through some other factor; 'substances in foods that also contain these nutrients, or a specific lifestyle may be responsible for the observed protective effect'. She is awaiting the results of controlled intervention trials to make her mind up.

6. 'Carotenoid Intake, Vegetables, and the Risk of Lung Cancer Among White Men in New Jersey', by Regina Ziegler *et al.*, *American Journal of Epidemiology*, vol. 123, no. 6, 1986, pp. 1080–93.

Ziegler's study was specifically targeted at lung cancer in high-risk areas of New Jersey. A retrospective dietary study, the research was aimed at finding out whether consumption of foods containing carotenoids, pre-formed vitamin A or total vitamin A had any influence over the risk of lung cancer.

The study looked at 763 cases and 900 controls. The cases were all men, aged 25 to 89 years, diagnosed with lung cancer between September 1, 1980 and October 31, 1981. Only those with cancer of the lung, no other part of the respiratory system, were analysed.

Each subject was interviewed and asked questions about tobacco use, diet, job, exposure to high-risk materials, residential and medical history. Dietary habits four years earlier were assessed by measuring the frequency of consumption of certain foods from a list of 44. The choice ranged from eggs, milk, cheese, butter, to carrots, green beans, asparagus, apricots and pink grapefruit. Those who were not sure what had been eaten or in what proportions were taken out of the analysis.

To gain an overall view, the average frequency of consumption over a whole year was calculated for each food item, and then the nutritional value of the food was analysed according to a typical portion. In this way the intake of pre-formed vitamin A, carotenoids, and total vitamin A intake, could be calculated.

Among the nutrients tested for, only carotenoids demonstrated an association with increased risk of lung cancer. No link could be found for vitamin A. The association seen in the following food groups: vegetables, dark green vegetables, dark yellow-orange vegetables, and vegetables and fruit, was even more striking than for carotenoids. Interestingly, low and moderate consumers of these food groups had a similar level of risk for developing lung cancer, when compared with high consumers; and the food group fruit seemed to make little difference.

This vegetable-related reduction in risk was seen in smokers of moderate and long duration, from which Ziegler concluded that vegetable intake could arrest the promotion of lung cancer rather than the initiation. Although the association was not particularly strong, it was consistent across all groups of people.

Ziegler concludes:

> Our case-control study suggests that carotenoids rather than total vitamin A are associated with a lowered risk of lung cancer and that consumption of vegetables, especially dark yellow-orange and dark-green vegetables, is even more predictive of reduced risk. The apparent protection by diet is most pronounced among current and recent cigarette smokers and smokers of long duration.[11]

7. 'Serum Beta-Carotene and Subsequent Risk of Cancer: Results from the BUPA Study', by Nicholas Wald et al., British Journal of Cancer, 57, 1988, pp. 428–33.

So far, this is the only big study to have come out of Britain. Commonly referred to as the BUPA Study, it was headed by

Professor Nicholas Wald of St Bartholomews Hospital in London. The aim of the research was to examine any connections between levels of beta-carotene in the blood and subsequent diagnosis of lung cancer.

The research took place on a massive scale, through the private health care scheme BUPA. Collection of blood samples from a total of 22,000 men, aged from 35 to 64, took place between 1975 and 1982. By April 1985, 271 men had developed cancer; two controls were chosen for each case, matched for age and smoking habits.

Overall, the average level of beta-carotene found in blood samples was lower in all cases of cancer than it was in controls. The cancers were divided into seven groups: lung, colorectal, stomach, bladder, central nervous system, skin and other. The lower levels were particularly significant in cancers of the lung and stomach.

Interestingly, Wald's results matched up with other studies: heavy smokers had the lowest beta-carotene levels. He was also able to conclude that the effect was present 'five and more years before the diagnosis of cancer . . . The low beta-carotene level probably precedes the development of cancer.'

8. 'Relationship Between Carotenoids and Cancer', by John Connett et al, Cancer 64, 1989, pp. 126–34.

The most recent research to be published on the association between nutrients and lung cancer is better known as the Multiple Risk Factor Intervention Trial study. The study is unique because it analysed blood levels of beta-carotene, total carotenoids, vitamin A, retinol binding protein (the protein to which vitamin A is attached and transported around the body), vitamin E and the mineral selenium.

There were 12,866 men involved in the study, between the ages of 35 and 57, all at high risk of coronary heart disease. At the outset, 63 per cent of the men were smokers, but they were all generally healthy, free of any cancers or coronary heart disease, and with no eating disorders.

Out of the chosen group of men, 156 developed cancer and to those were assigned 311 controls. Among the 66 cases of lung cancer the blood levels of total carotenoids were significantly lower when compared to their controls, and the beta-carotene was slightly lower. Like Gey and the Basel Study (below), Connett stated that he did not believe an undetected cancer had effected the lower levels of carotenoids and beta-carotene. In his conclusion he wrote:

> Our results are consistent with the National Cancer Institute's recent recommendation for increased consumption of green and yellow vegetables . . . we conclude that the possible link between lung cancer and beta-carotene, other carotenoids, and other nutrients found in green or yellow vegetables is highly deserving of further evaluation and research.

Lung and Stomach

1. 'Plasma Levels of Antioxidant Vitamins in Relation to Ischemic Heart Disease and Cancer', by Gey *et al.*, *American Journal of Clinical Nutrition*, 45, 1987, pp. 1368–77.

This study had two prongs of attack: ischemic heart disease (when there is a shortage of blood to the heart usually caused by thickening of the artery walls) and cancer. Gey and colleagues wanted to find out whether antioxidant nutrients (see Chapter 8), vitamins A, C, E and beta-carotene, had any effect on the risk of developing either of these conditions.

The cancer part of the research programme is better known in medical circles as the Basel study. It was a prospective study which began with 3,000 apparently healthy men, all employees of pharmaceutical companies based in Basel, Switzerland. Their average age was 51 and they had their blood measured for the above vitamins between the years of 1971 and 1973.

The researchers were involved in a seven-year follow-up period and found that beta-carotene levels in cases diagnosed with lung and stomach cancer were significantly lower than those of other members of the study without these cancers. A significant decrease in vitamin A and beta-carotene was linked to stomach cancer. In general, levels of vitamins C, E and beta-carotene, were decreased for all major cancer types. Gey suggested: 'The data of the Basel Study suggest an organ-specific risk pattern of the essential antioxidants.'

Interestingly, Gey also proposed the idea that these nutrients worked in synergy. For example in stomach cancer, if low levels of both beta-carotene and vitamin A occurred simultaneously the risk of stomach cancer almost doubled. He writes: 'A potential preventive effect of vitamin A may thus require an optimal status of beta-carotene and vice versa'. Other connections linking the protective effect of the nutrients were noticed for beta-carotene and vitamin C in stomach cancer, and for beta-carotene and vitamin E in lung cancer.

Like the researchers before him, Gey ends on a cautionary note, reminding us that 'Even the hardest epidemiological [statistical] evidence cannot prove any causal relationship between essential antioxidants and mortality . . . the other dietary components (minerals, fibres etc) remain to be excluded.'

Stomach

1. 'Diet in the Epidemiology of Gastric Cancer', Saxon Graham *et al.*, *Nutrition and Cancer*, 13, 1990, pp. 19–34.

Graham and colleagues were keen to analyse why certain ethnic groups should suffer more stomach cancer, and why there had been such a steep decline generally in the number of cases diagnosed. They already knew that diets low in carotenoids, vitamins A and C, raw vegetables and high in salt, nitrates, meats and fats had shown a statistical link with the incidence of stomach cancer.

For their participants, the Graham team drew on stomach cancer cases in the west of New York state. They researched the diets and lifestyles of 293 patients (men and women), selected over a ten-year period (1975 to 1985).

The study found that the risk of stomach cancer in those who had a high intake of carotenoids was significantly less than those who ate far fewer sources of the nutrient. It was also able to isolate certain significant vegetables: for men they were celery, cucumber, carrots, green peppers, tomatoes and onions; for women, onions and winter squash (a large gourd commonly eaten in the USA). Higher intake of raw vegetables also showed a protective link.

Graham concluded:

> Limiting caloric intake, especially fat, limiting sodium, and increasing vegetable intake, particularly vegetables containing carotene, are suggested steps toward inhibiting the risk of stomach cancer ... A number of other cancers (e.g. colon and lung) in addition to cardiovascular pathologies [heart disease] might also be controlled by these dietary suggestions.

Mouth

1. 'Reduction with Vitamin A and Beta-Carotene Administration of Proportion of Micronucleated Buccal Mucosal Cells in Asian Betel Nut and Tobacco Chewers', by Hans Stich et al., The Lancet, June 2, 1984, pp. 1204–6.

Stich has carried out a number of 'intervention' trials with beta-carotene and vitamin A to find out whether they can reduce the occurrence of mouth cancer. Every year in Asia mouth cancer causes several hundred thousand deaths;[12] the main reason for this is the traditional habit of chewing betel nuts. These are carcinogenic, and can cause harm to the DNA of mouth cells.

Often people will be chewing up to 15 'quids' of betel nut every day. Betel nut chewers tend to be poor people, and it is quite a task to convince them of the dangers inherent in chewing. The 'micronucleated' cells mentioned in the title of the study enclose damaged pieces of DNA. The damage occurs when the cell is replaced with a new one. The introduction of a carcinogen such as betel nut can increase the damage by up to ten times.

The formation of micronuclei does not mean that cancer has

taken hold, but it can indicate a change in the cells that could in turn lead to cancer. In their study, Stich and colleagues looked at whether supplementation with a mixture of beta-carotene and vitamin A could have an effect on the formation of these micronuclei.

The setting for the study was the Philippines, the participants were chosen from the Ifugaos hill tribe in northern Luzon. A total of 40 men and women aged between 30 and 60 were chosen for the investigation. They were all daily chewers, consuming up to 15 quids a day for an average of 12 minutes each.

The daily diet of the participants was very poor, consisting of rice and sweet potatoes, a few boiled taro leaves and a handful of cow peas. Consumption of fruit and meat was rare; and none of the volunteers smoked tobacco.

Over a period of three months, the Philippino men and women were administered two capsules of vitamin A (100,000 IU) and 6 capsules of beta-carotene (300,000 IU) every week. The capsules were swallowed whole, and did not come into contact with the inside of the mouth.

At the beginning and the end of the trial, exfoliated cells from the inner lining of the mouth were scraped off and examined. Initially the betel nut chewers had high levels of micronuclei visible in their inner cheek samples, but this manifestation was greatly reduced three months later, after the supplementation. Professor Stich concluded that if micronuclei were proved to have a link with oral cancer, 'then our data suggest that some people at high risk of oral cancer may be able to modify those risks by nutritional supplement.'

More recent work by Stich and Professor Harinder Garewal has shown that the development of leukoplakia, the pre-cancerous stage of mouth cancer, can be reversed with supplements of vitamin A and beta-carotene.[3,4] Stich showed that vitamin A was initially more effective than beta-carotene at reducing oral leukoplakia, but suggested that maintenance doses of beta-carotene could keep the leukoplakia at bay. In a study carried out on Indian fishermen who chewed betel quids, the micronuclei and leukoplakias reappeared after supplementation with the two nutrients was stopped. In studies carried out by Professor Garewal at the University of Arizona, results have suggested that beta-carotene on its own can reverse oral leukoplakia in 70 per cent of patients. More research by different sicentists is needed fully to validate the proposals put forward by Stich and Garewal.

Minor Studies

The links between beta-carotene and lung cancer are the most prominent, with mouth cancer showing a lot of promise. But there have also been a number of smaller studies looking at cancers of the breast, prostate and cervix.

The breast cancer study[5] was based in Adelaide, South Australia and examined the links found between the disease and diet. Dietary intake was measured by food frequency questionnaires. The study did not support any significant risk factor for levels of fat, protein, sugar, starch, or vitamin A, but did show a protective link from intake of beta-carotene. It concludes: 'The study has provided evidence that suggests an inverse association between the level of beta-carotene in the diet and risk of breast cancer.'

The study related to prostate cancer[6] was again a case-control dietary study of 371 prostate cancer patients admitted to a hospital in Buffalo, New York. The organizers set out to discover whether levels of dietary animal fats and green and yellow vegetables had any effect on prostate cancer.

The researchers found that young men in particular had a reduced risk of developing the cancer if they had a high intake of beta-carotene, but added:

> When these findings are evaluated with those of other recent investigations on diet and prostate cancer, no consistent pattern of findings for beta-carotene and risk can be established . . . The available data probably do not allow any conclusions on the nature of the association between beta-carotene and prostate cancer risk.

The final study of interest was aimed at researching the effects of nutrients in cervical cancer.[7] This was another Australian trial, based in Sydney. It looked at 117 women with cervical cancer, investigating vitamin A status, number of sexual partners, age at first intercourse, smoking and oral contraceptive use.

The research team found that dietary intake of fruit juices, salad vegetables and soups was significantly related to risk. The consumption of fruits did not appear to lower the risk. The paper concluded:

> No nutrient shows a clear effect, although vitamin C is the most likely candidate despite the fact that fruits were not associated with reduced risk. High levels of blood carotenoids, however, were protective, especially beta-carotene.

Conclusion

All the three studies mentioned above show a positive effect of beta-carotene on other cancers and yet scientists remain unconvinced. The strongest protective link with cancer is without doubt that between beta-carotene and lung cancer, particularly the squamous cell type.

Much work remains to be done, but a huge amount of interest has been generated by existing research; enough to sponsor upwards of seven intervention trials on the beneficial effects of supplementation with beta-carotene (either via food or a capsule). Intervention trials currently running (described at greater length in Chapter 11) include those looking at cancers of the lung, skin and all sites. The results are waited upon with bated breath by many in the field, who feel beta-carotene and possibly other carotenoids have a valuable part to play in protecting the body against the invasion of cancer.

Notes

1. Parkin, D.M., 'Estimates of the worldwide frequency of 12 major cancers', *Bulletin of World Health Organization*, 1984.

2. Stich, H.F., 'Beta-carotene levels in exfoliated mucosa cells of population groups at low and elevated risk of oral cancer', *International Journal of Cancer*, 1986, 37, pp. 389–93.
3. *Ibid*.
4. Stich, H. *et al.*, 'Human intervention studies with carotenoids', *8th International Symnposium on Carotenoids*, Boston, MA, abstract No. 45.
5. Rohan, T.E. *et al.*, 'A population-based case-control study of diet and breast cancer in Australia', *American Journal of Epidemiology*, 128, no. 3.
6. Mettlin, C. *et al.*, 'Beta-carotene and animal fats and the relationship to prostate cancer risk', *Cancer*, 64, 1989, pp. 605–12.
7. Brock, K.E. *et al.*, 'Nutrients in diet and plasma and risk of in situ cervical cancer', *Journal of the National Cancer Institute*, June 15, 1988, 80, pp. 580–5.

Chapter 8

Beta-Carotene vs Cancer – How Could it Work?

In the last two chapters we have read that a high proportion of cancers could be caused by outside influences; and that dietary components such as fat, fibre and nutrients could also have significant influence over the development of the disease. Beta-carotene, in particular, has been singled out to be investigated for its protective role against cancer.

Scientists know that beta-carotene is not just able to form vitamin A inside the body, but it is also an effective antioxidant and a quencher of singlet oxygen. Vitamin A does not possess those qualities. Because of this it is believed that beta-carotene may have a protective role to play in its own right, a role which according to American scientist, Dr Adrianne Bendich, could protect DNA strands from initial mutation, or slow down the promotion stage of cancer, thus lessening the tumour burden.

Studies linking vitamin A and its precursor beta-carotene with cancer prevention have been going on for many years; vitamin A may have an effect because of its role in controlling cell proliferation, but it is only recently that scientists have begun to analyse how beta-carotene, as an independent nutrient, could protect against cancer. Even so, some scientists, such as Dr Bendich, think that beta-carotene's vitamin A capacity could work in synergy with the other aspects of the nutrient.

To put the research into context, it is important to remember that cancer is a multi-faceted condition, which is still not fully understood. There are obvious difficulties involved in under-standing how intervention in a disease works when the disease itself is not clearly mapped out; it is a little like pinning a tail onto a donkey, blindfold.

Added to the confusion are the five or six 'alternative' carotenoids that have not been investigated to anything like the extent of beta-carotene. Carotenoids like lycopene, lutein and cryptoxanthin are major players in the dietary field. Dr Regina Ziegler, of the US National Cancer Institute (NCI) reminds us that only beta-carotene has been fully investigated. Over the next few years the NCI will be researching into these three carotenoids, as well as alpha-carotene. Dr David Thurnham of the Dunn Nutrition Centre, Cambridge, is also very interested in these other major carotenoids.

The Potential of Beta-Carotene

Until more research on the carotenoid family has been done, beta-carotene remains the nutrient about which most is known. So, just why could beta-carotene by any different from any other substance? First, as an antioxidant it can mop up free radicals; second, it is the most efficient quencher of singlet oxygen known; and third, both these properties may enhance the day-to-day business of the human immune system.

Antioxidants and Free Radicals

Free radicals are highly reactive molecules which can damage the internal structure of the body. They are reactive because they are one electron short (electrons like to be in pairs) and will grab an electron from another molecule, so creating a chain of imbalance and causing cellular disruption. They can also be found in food, and cause oxidation, making wine, cheese or butter for example, go off.

A molecule is made from atoms; atoms contain electrons, little energy packs, which are the basis of all living things. An ion is an electrically-charged particle, resulting from the breakdown of atoms in water.

In the human body, free radicals are naturally occurring – an essential intermediate of the body's normal defence mechanisms against disease. However, they can also be 'baddies' when formed by external factors such as smoke, tar, pesticides, and certain drugs such as paracetamol. Some carcinogens such as X-rays can provoke the creation of free radicals.

Antioxidants are substances which can quench free radicals and stop them from doing any damage. They do this by donating an electron and simply decaying harmlessly afterwards. Antioxidants are obtained from the food we eat, notably vitamins C and E, beta-carotene and the mineral selenium. They are also made in the body as enzymes, notably glutathione peroxidase, catalase and superoxide dismutase, which sit inside cells waiting to detoxify the reactive free radicals.

Since the early 1970s[1] the free radical theory of disease has been steadily gaining more credence in the scientific world. The effects of free radical damage have been linked with the following medical conditions: radiation injury, disease of the retina, cataracts, rheumatoid arthritis, Alzheimer's disease (nervous dementia), ischaemic heart disease, atherosclerosis, some forms of cancer, and premature ageing. The latest strand of research is looking at the generation of free radicals in organs undergoing transfusion. It appears that the free radical theory of disease is filling in some of the gaps left by previous medical research.

How do Free Radicals Work?

Free radicals are able to upset the equilibrium of other cellular constituents because their habit of electron-grabbing or donating causes a chain reaction; as soon as one molecule is one electron short, it will steal another and so on. But, the first thing to recognize, says Dr Catherine Rice-Evans of St Thomas's Hospital Medical School – a leading British authority on free radicals – is that they are not totally destructive, but play a very important part of our normal defence against bacteria.

So, some free radicals are 'goodies'! Neutrophils are cells

which are an essential part of our defence system; when bacteria invade the body, neutrophils are activated and try to repel the bacteria, and as a weapon they produce superoxide free radicals. If you damage your skin, you will notice an inflammation occurring – this involves the action of your body's neutrophils and the superoxide radicals which they produce.

In short-term health conditions this resonse is fine, but in long-term chronic disease states, such as rheumatoid arthritis, superoxide radicals continue to be generated by the neutrophils and can overload the body's antioxidant quenchers, which means the situation worsens. This is when internally-produced free radicals, essential to our defences, can be dangerous – when produced in excess of normal requirements.

In general, superoxide radicals are quenched by the antioxidant enzyme superoxide dismutase, which is found in every cell. This changes superoxide radicals into hydrogen peroxide – a 'reactive oxygen species' but not a free radical. Hydrogen peroxide has the ability to move around the body and enter cells, and it can arrive at sites closed off to many other substances. Added to this is its ability to form the highly toxic free radical hydroxyl, if it meets a molecule of iron or copper.

Normally, iron is not freely available in the body. However in certain diseases it may become delocalized and bleed into the joints (e.g. in rheumatoid arthritis). In this form it can help to form toxic free radicals and is able to combine with hydrogen peroxide to make a hydroxyl radical. The hydroxyl radical is so reactive it will react with the first thing it meets and, because it can be inside a cell, it is capable of damaging DNA.

Hydrogen peroxide molecules can be quenched by the enzyme antioxidant glutathione peroxidase or by another anti-oxidant called catalase. However, glutathione peroxidase is dependent on the micronutrient selenium; so if you have low levels of this, your inbuilt antioxidants may not work very well.

Superoxide free radicals can also be formed when there is a disruption of the process in the mitochondria, the part of the cell which turns oxygen into water. Other free radicals are formed by external factors such as cigarette smoke and certain drugs.

All these free radicals have to go somewhere, and their effects are not limited to one reaction. Whatever they react with, they will in turn look for another electron to pair with from a different molecule, what Dr Rice-Evans terms the 'ricochet effect'. At some stage the free radical will be quenched by an antioxidant or will simply peter out. If there is no antioxidant available, one free radical could, by this means, destroy the functioning of the whole cell and membrane. Incidentally, all these reactions happen in the space of a split second and are going on all the time.

What do Free Radicals Damage?
Free radicals disable lipids, the fatty substances that form membranes (blubbery marine animals have many lipids); proteins (the body's building blocks and enzymes); and DNA. If free radicals steal electrons from these components they can cause disruption to cell walls, causing leakage of the cells to sites where their contents should not be; they damage organelles (microscopic 'organs' inside cells); cause mutation in DNA; and they damage enzymes (proteins that facilitate all bodily functions).[2]

For example, lipids are found in the membranes surrounding cells. The membranes act as a type of bag around the cell, keeping all the important things safely inside. If a free radical attacks a lipid belonging to a membrane, the membrane can become leaky and the things inside can start to leak out. Equally unhealthy are damaged enzymes, because if they are not working properly all sorts of tiny but vital reactions will be affected. This response could be significant in the promotion stage of cancer.

Antioxidant Quenchers
When any kind of free radical is generated in the body – be it from external or internal causes – there is an antidote available; an antioxidant, so called because they prevent further oxidation.

Enzymes
According to Professor Anthony Diplock of Guy's Hospital,

London, the first level of antioxidant defence is enzymic, involving mainly glutathione peroxidase and superoxide dismutase. These are formed from a variety of micronutrients such as manganese, copper, zinc and selenium. If your body's stocks of these are low, then your defences will be low. These antioxidants lie inside the cells.

Nutrients

The second level of defence, if free radicals manage to avoid the important enzymes, comes from the vitamins E, C and beta-carotene. By eating foods rich in these nutrients the body is stocked up with efficient antioxidants. These nutrient antioxidants are found outside the cell as well as inside. Vitamin E is found in all cell membranes, in lipoproteins, and in the blood plasma. Vitamin C is one of the most important antioxidants inside blood plasma. And beta-carotene is found in the core of the lipoproteins. These nutrients are, in the words of Professor John Marks, 'a vital aspect of antioxidant defence.'[3]

Vitamin E is the major fat-soluble antioxidant, and can react directly with peroxyl and hydroxyl radicals by giving them a spare electron. In other words it can stop damage to membrane lipids and lipoproteins begun by damage caused by free radicals. Vitamin E can be regenerated by vitamin C, and protects vitamin A and beta-carotene from oxidation in humans.[4] Vitamin E seems to be the prime antioxidant which scavenges free radicals, itself being regenerated by 'helper' antioxidants like vitamin C, so that vitamin E can carry on with its work without being used up too rapidly.

Beta-Carotene

Beta-carotene acts as an antioxidant and also as a powerful quencher of singlet oxygen. It is particularly good at quenching peroxyl free radicals involved in attacking lipids. Dr Catherine Rice-Evans has described experiments in which blood is taken from patients and the lipoproteins separated. Then a substance is added to introduce free radicals, and using a special instrument you can see beta-carotene disappearing as it quenches the free radicals. Beta-carotene needs a lot of topping up to maintain normal healthy levels.

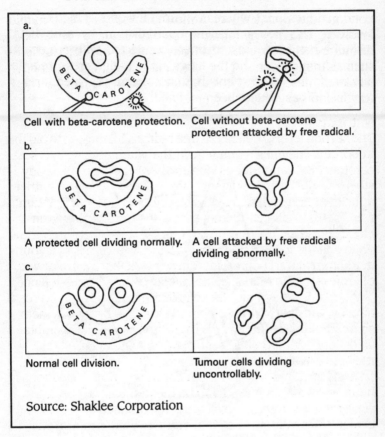

a.

Cell with beta-carotene protection.   Cell without beta-carotene protection attacked by free radical.

b.

A protected cell dividing normally.   A cell attacked by free radicals dividing abnormally.

c.

Normal cell division.   Tumour cells dividing uncontrollably.

Source: Shaklee Corporation

Figure 8.1: Beta-carotene as an antioxidant.

Beta-carotene molecules are relatively low in numbers; their concentration is much lower than that of vitamin E. For each lipoprotein there are eleven molecules of vitamin E, but there is only one beta-carotene molecule for every three lipoproteins. According to Dr David Thurnham of the Dunn Nutrition Centre, Cambridge, carotenoids also need to be protected by other antioxidants, or they are oxidized and lost during absorption.

One study made on beta-carotene's capability as an antioxidant shows how it appears to work much better at low levels of oxygen pressure,[5] whereas vitamin E works at high oxygen pressure. This poses a slight contradiction, because beta-carotene has been most strongly connected with protection against lung cancer and the lungs are in a high pressure area. However, this experiment has not been repeated and a conclusion has not yet been reached.

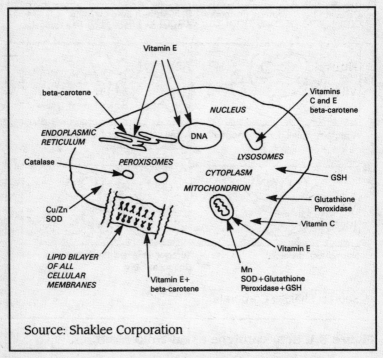

Source: Shaklee Corporation

Figure 8.2: Antioxidant protection within the cell.

Dr Graham Burton, of the National Research Council of Canada, suggests that the explanation for beta-carotene's protective effect as an antioxidant is tenuous. He has put forward another way that beta-carotene could work – because it is very sensitive to oxidation itself, the end-products could be toxic to cancer cells. Dr Burton freely admits he has no proof for this and is just throwing the idea out, but it does serve to remind us that the effects of beta-carotene still pose many questions.

Working in Synergy

As research continues it is widely believed that in order to work efficiently, the antioxidants must work together. They have synergistic qualities, which means that they complement one another. If you only ever ate foods containing beta-carotene, you would not be getting the full benefits of its ability to be an antioxidant; the same with vitamins C, E, and selenium. To recommend one without the others is shortsighted.

Nutrient	Activity
Vitamin C (ascorbic acid)	Important water-soluble cytosolic chain-breaking antioxidant: reacts directly with superoxide, singlet oxygen; regenerates tocopherol from tocopheroxy radical
Vitamin E (alpha-tocopherol)	Major membrane-bound, lipid-soluble chain-breaking antioxidant; reacts directly with superoxide, singlet oxygen
Beta-carotene	Most potent singlet oxygen quencher, antioxidant properties particularly at low oxygen pressure, lipid soluble
Zinc	Constituent of cytosolic superoxide dismutase
Selenium	Constituent of glutathione peroxidase
Copper	Constituent of cytosolic superoxide dismutase and ceruloplasmin

Nutrient	Activity
Iron	Constituent of catalase
Manganese	Constituent of mitochondrial superoxide dismutase

Source: Shaklee Corporation

Table 8.3: Antioxidant micronutrients

Beta-Carotene as a Quencher of Singlet Oxygen

Beta-carotene is the most efficient quencher of singlet oxygen known. The oxygen we normally breathe is called triplet state oxygen, and is very stable. Singlet oxygen is generated when there is a sudden burst of energy and it immediately becomes unstable and excitable. In order to become stable again (which all chemicals want to do) it must react chemically with something else, and this can cause damage.

Fortunately, singlet oxygen is not that common compared with free radicals, and does not act as such a major catalyst when looking at the causes of disease. However, it is not to be discounted, and can create toxic reactions within cells in order to return to its normal low energy state. In this context, beta-carotene's role as an active and successful quencher is very useful.

Beta-Carotene and the Immune System

Beta-carotene's function as an antioxidant is also thought to play a significant role in keeping the immune system fit and healthy.[6] Exactly how it does this is not yet firmly established, but beta-carotene would certainly stop free radicals from damaging any of the white blood cells involved in defending our bodies from foreign materials in our bloodstream and tissues.

Dr Bendich points out that beta-carotene could have different effects on different cancers, and that in some cases beta-carotene is protective in pre-cancerous states such as oral leukoplakia (the white spots inside the mouth which indicate a possible cancerous state). In other cancers it could be protective in that it slows down the rate of tumour growth, or stops free radical damage. An effect of bolstering up the immune system could work in either the initiation or the promotion stage, 'At this stage we cannot make generalizations', says Dr Bendich.

To date, the research showing the beta-carotene/immune system boost has been done mostly on cell cultures and animal models (rats and mice). Yet this type of work shows potential for human application. A recent paper written by Professor Krinsky of Tufts University, Boston,[7] summarized the cell culture and rodent tests, which showed how beta-carotene could protect against UV-light induced skin cancers by slowing the growth rate of tumours, and reducing the levels of colon cancer. In the abstract of his paper, Professor Krinsky writes:

> Observations have been made in cell and organ cultures where carotenoids have been shown to prevent malignant transformation and nuclear damage. Although the mechanism of this protection is still unclear, the evidence continues to accumulate that carotenoids may possess intrinsic chemopreventive action with respect to tumour formation.

He cautions that, although these kind of controlled laboratory tests demonstrate a protective function, they require further evidence before the information can be 'applicable to human studies'. Even so, two human intervention trials are looking at beta-carotene in relation to skin cancer (one on albinos, one on subjects with basal cell carcinoma).

As an immunologist, Dr Bendich spends much of her time examining the details of beta-carotene's capabilities. In a 1988 paper she writes that there is growing evidence that beta-carotene can boost immune protection.[8] This is true not just for beta-carotene, but also for other members of the carotenoid family such as bixin, canthaxanthin, astaxanthin and alpha-carotene; these have antioxidant and singlet oxygen quenching functions too, opening up a 'new frontier for carotenoid research'.

Bendich reiterates the observation that superoxide radicals, produced by neutrophils to kill off bacteria, can be over-produced, and therefore be damaging to neighbouring tissue and neutrophils. When human neutrophils were incubated with beta-carotene and bacteria, the bacteria were killed off, but the superoxide radicals did not damage the neutrophils. To contrast with these results, neutrophils and bacteria incubated without beta-carotene were damaged by superoxide free radicals.

Other cells involved in the immune response can be damaged as a result of free radicals,[9,10,11,12] and studies have shown that vitamin A and beta-carotene can both increase the number of lymphocytes and T cells (a sub-group of lymphocytes).[13,14] It has also been shown that damage to macrophages (white blood cells which recognize bacteria) could be inhibited by beta-carotene and canthaxanthin after exposure to substances which are not free radicals, but which can turn into them.[15]

Another study observed that T helper cells in humans were significantly increased when patients were supplemented with beta-carotene for two weeks (180 milligrams a day).[16] To prove that the effect was due to the independent capabilities of beta-carotene, rather than vitamin A, a further study was carried out using beta-carotene and canthaxanthin.[17] Canthaxanthin has the same antioxidant and singlet oxygen quenching abilities as beta-carotene, but cannot be made into vitamin A. Both carotenoids enhanced immune response.

There have been other studies which show that the cell types capable of killing tumour cells – namely macrophages, natural killer cells and cytotoxic T cells – can have their actions enhanced by beta-carotene;[18,19,20,21] and that mice given beta-carotene developed smaller tumours than mice which were not.[22]

There remains much research to be done in order to establish whether it is beta-carotene, or something else in fruit and vegetables, that shows a protective effect against cancers. The

Carotenoid	Effect
Beta-carotene	Prevented stress-induced thymic involution and lymphopenia
Beta-carotene	Increased graft vs host response
Beta-carotene, bixin	Enhanced regression of virally-induced tumours
Beta-carotene	Increased helper T lymphocytes (human beings)
Beta-carotene, canthaxanthin	Enhanced T and B cell proliferation
Beta-carotene, canthaxanthin, astaxanthin, phycotene (algae extract)	Increased cytotoxic macrophage and T cell activities in tumour models
Beta-carotene, beta-carotene + canthaxanthin	Maintained macrophage receptors for antigens
Beta-carotene, alpha-carotene	Increased natural killer cell lysis of tumour cells

Source: A. Bendich, Clinical Nutrition

Figure 8.4: Evidence for carotenoid immunoenhancement.

priority for scientists is to demonstrate the mechanisms of action in humans, rather than cell cultures, mice and rats. Whether beta-carotene works against the initiation or the promotion of cancer, depends on the type of cancer and the carcinogenic agent(s). What we can be sure of is that the research work done thus far will lead to an even greater understanding of how we might conquer cancer.

Notes

1. Slater, T.F., 'Free Radical Mechanism in Tissue Injury', Pion, London, 1972.
2. Marks, J., 'Clinical implications of free radicals', *Naringsforskning*, 33, 1989, pp. 130–7.
3. *Ibid*.
4. Freeman, B.A. and Crapo, J.D., 'Biology of disease: free radicals and tissue injury', *Laboratory Investigation*, 47, 1982, pp. 412–26.
5. Burton, G.W. and Ingold, K.U., 'Beta-carotene – an unusual type of lipid antioxidant', *Science*, 224, 1984, pp. 569–73.
6. Bendich, A., 'Carotenoids and the immune response', *Journal of Nutrition*, 119, 1, 1989, pp. 112–5.
7. Krinsky, N.I., 'Carotenoids and cancer in animal models', *Journal of Nutrition*, 119, 1, 1989, pp. 123–6.
8. See 6.
9. Mertin, J. and Hunt, R., 'Influence of polyunsaturated fatty acids on survival of skin allografts and tumour incidence on mice', *Proceedings of the National Academy of Science, USA*, 73, 1976, pp. 928–31.
10. Erickson, K.L. *et al.*, 'Influence of dietary fat concentration and saturation on immune ontogeny in mice', *Journal of Nutrition*, 110, 1980, pp. 1555–72.
11. Newberne, P.M., 'Dietary fat, immunological response and cancer in rats', *Cancer Research*, 41, 1981, pp. 3783–5.
12. Gurr, M.I., 'The role of lipids in the regulation of the immune system', *Progress in Lipid Research*, 22, 1983, pp. 257–87.
13. Seifter, E. *et al.*, 'Carotenoids and cell-mediated immune responses', in Charalambors, G., and Inglett, G. (eds.), *The Quality of Foods and Beverages*, Academic Press, New York, 1981, pp. 335–47.
14. Seifter, E. *et al.*, 'Moloney murine sarcoma virus tumours in CBA/J mice: chemopreventive and chemotherapeutic actions of supplemental beta-carotene', *Journal of the National Cancer Institute*, 68, 1982, pp. 835–40.
15. Gruner, S. *et al.*, 'The influence of phagocytic stimuli on the expression of HLA-DR antigens; role of reactive oxygen intermediates', *European Journal of Immunology*, 6, 1986, pp. 212–5.

16. Alexander, M. *et al.*, 'Oral beta-carotene can increase the number of OKT4+ cells in human blood', *Immunology Letters*, 9, 1985, 221–4.
17. Bendich, A. and Shapiro, S.S., 'Effect of beta-carotene and canthaxanthin on the immune responses of the rat', *Journal of Nutrition*, 116, 1986, pp. 2254–62.
18. Leslie, C.A. and Dubey, D.P., 'Carotene and natural killer cell activity', *Federal Proceedings*, 41, 1982, p. 331.
19. Schwartz, J. *et al.*, 'Beta-carotene is associated with the regression of hamster buccal pouch carcinoma and the induction of tumour necrosis factor in macrophages', *Biochemical and Biophysical Research Committee*, 136, 1986, pp. 1130–5.
20. Shklar, G. and Schwartz, J., 'Tumour necrosis factor in experimental cancer regression with vitamin E, beta-carotene, canthaxanthin and algae extract'. *European Journal of Cancer*, 1988, 24(5), pp. 839–50.
21. Schwartz, J. and Shklar, G., 'Regression of experimental hamster cancer by beta-carotene and algae extracts', *Oral Maxillofacial Surgery Clinics of North America*, 45, 1987, pp. 510–5.
22. Tomita, Y. *et al.*, 'Augmentation of tumour immunity against syngenic tumours in mice by beta-carotene', *Journal of the National Cancer Institute*, 78, 1987, pp. 679–80.

Chapter 9

Other Potential Roles for Beta-Carotene

The current research into the role beta-carotene can play in health matters is not confined simply to cancer – work has been initiated in other areas too. The main alternative fields of interest are cataracts, heart disease and other diseases involving free radicals. As yet, there is little concrete evidence to go on in these areas, but enough to continue research.

Cataracts

Cataracts tend to occur in the elderly, and can also be a result of diabetes. The pupil and iris of the eye become clouded over and opaque, causing dimness of vision. Scientists believe that free radicals could play a part in the formation of cataracts. Inside the eye the role of the lens is to collect and focus light on the retina, as a result it is permanently subjected to photo-oxidative stress. Cataracts may appear mainly in old age because by this time the eye has been put under many years of such stress, and the development of free radicals and singlet oxygen may have occurred. As explained in Chapter 8, these unbalanced substances can cause damage to cells and tissues.

As usual, however, the body has its own defence system against these potentially damaging elements. One system is comprised of specialized enzymes which deactivate free radicals; these include superoxide dismutase, catalase and glutathione peroxidase. The second line of defence uses vitamin C, vitamin E and beta-carotene to quench free radicals and singlet oxygen.

Vitamin C has a particularly high concentration in the lens, and the rods and cones of the eye contain the specific carotenoids, lutein and zeaxanthin. (These are derived from alpha- and beta-carotene.) All the antioxidants help to support and regenerate one another if they are present in sufficient quantities.

The same role beta-carotene plays in plants may be involved in its protection of the eye. It protects plants from light damage by quenching singlet oxygen, and could do similar things inside the eye. Although more research is required, the hypothesis is that beta-carotene could act as a light filter within the eye.

Patients with the skin condition erythropoietic proto-porphyria (EPP) are treated effectively with mega-doses of beta-carotene, because it is able to quench the singlet oxygen generated by the patient's abnormal reaction to sunlight. Such well-documented success implies that it is quite possible for beta-carotene to work against other pockets of singlet oxygen in the body.

One scientific study has looked into the relationship between nutrition and senile cataracts.[1] The nutritional status and levels of cataract were examined in 112 subjects aged between 40 and 70. Seventy-seven of the participants in the study had a cataract in at least one lens. The nutrients measured included total carotenoids, vitamin A, vitamin C, vitamin D, vitamin E, magnesium, selenium and zinc.

The most striking finding of the study was a strong association of risk between low vitamin D and development of cataracts. People with cataracts tended to go out into the sunshine less, and vitamin D is manufactured from sunshine. Another interesting observation was that participants with high or moderate carotenoid levels had a lower risk of developing cataracts. The other nutrients were also found to play an important role in protection against cataracts.

The study concludes:

Evidence suggests that nutritional status may influence cataract occurrence in humans. The possible nutritional determinants identified in this analysis are consistent with the hypothesis that cataract formation may be delayed by the lens antioxidants and accelerated by the presence of oxidants, although this hypothesis may not be sufficient to explain all of our results.

Heart Disease

There are several forms of heart disease, and by far the most common one is called atherosclerosis. Over years, a build-up of greasy material, mainly cholesterol, lines the walls of the arteries (the thick tubes which carry blood away from the heart). As the greasy layers build up, the arteries can cope with less blood, and therefore the heart is put under strain. Results can be thrombosis (an abnormal blood clot), which, in the brain, causes a stroke, or in the heart causes coronary thrombosis. Angina – when the heart does not function efficiently – can also occur, as can a general lack of efficiency in the muscles, the kidneys and the rest of the body, because of low blood supply. If the blood supply to the kidneys is threatened, blood pressure rises to compensate and aggravates the atherosclerosis.

Over the last decade, the discovery that cholesterol is largely responsible for atherosclerosis has given this substance a very bad image. The truth is that cholesterol is essential to bodily health, found in the cells and blood of all animals. We don't have to eat cholesterol to maintain levels, because the body already makes it within the liver.

Chemically, cholesterol is completely water insoluble, and therefore cannot pass through cell walls under its own steam. Instead the body has to supply it with a means of transport. These transporters come in the form of tiny particles known as low-density lipoproteins (LDLs).

All is well until, on top of the cholesterol our bodies produce, we start to consume an excess of dietary saturated (animal) fats which contain high levels of cholesterol. The LDLs cannot cope with so much cholesterol, and begin to run out of places to put it. At this stage they start to dump it in the arteries.

The natural safety net against this occurring is a related group of substances known as high-density lipoproteins (or

HDLs). The function of HDLs is to scavenge 'dumped' cholesterol from the tissues and return it to the liver for disposal. People with low HDL counts are more at risk from heart disease, and therefore a heart attack. Eating fish oils, which contain fatty acids, increases the level of HDL in the blood and is thought to lower risk. Some people inherit low levels of HDL and tend to be at a greater risk of heart disease.

Essential fatty acids from fish oils can help lower the risk of heart disease by creating higher levels of HDLs as opposed to LDLs; but new research suggests that LDLs can cause even more damage if they are oxidized by free radicals (see Chapter 8). When a low-density lipoprotein is oxidized, its form is changed, and it is no longer recognized by the cell to which it is delivering the cholesterol. Instead of going to its proper destination, the changed LDL is swept up by scavenging cells called macrophages, and turned into foam cells. These cells still contain the cholesterol, but have jagged edges and grip onto the side of arteries, causing the fatty streaks of atherosclerosis.[2,3]

This is where the antioxidant nutrients can save the day. Within a molecule of LDL there are several different components, including vitamin E, beta-carotene and lycopene, which protect the molecule from oxidation. Under test circumstances it has been shown that if LDL is subject to oxidative substances, the antioxidants present in the LDL get used up quickly. This suggests that a supply of antioxidants is needed to quell oxidation, but more human research is needed before it can be shown without doubt that antioxidants can lower the risk of atherosclerosis, through protecting LDL. A study looking at the levels of antioxidants in lipoproteins is currently under way at the London Chest Hospital. When lipoproteins are isolated in a test tube and subjected to free radical attack, the beta-carotene disappears very quickly, while the vitamin E stays intact longer.

Recent results from a large-scale intervention trial called the Hennekens Trial (see Chapter 11) have shown that men taking 50 mg of beta-carotene every other day have a just under 50 per cent reduction in all major areas of coronary ill health, compared with the control group. This is the most specific research available about beta-carotene and heart disease, and suggests a tremendous potential for its use in 'at risk' patients.

Transplantation

The use of antioxidants during organ transplantation is another growing area of research. For example, when a kidney is taken from a donor it must be stored and preserved in some way before being re-implanted. When the organ is transplanted into a new body, it is reperfused with oxygen to bring it back to life – at this point free radicals can be created. Treatment of the organ with antioxidants could be used to stop the free radicals being generated, ensuring better preservation and viability for transplantation. Beta-carotene, along with other antioxidants, could have an important role to play here.

Notes

1. Jacques, P.F. and Hartz, S.C., 'Nutritional status in persons with and without senile cataract: blood vitamin and mineral levels', *American Journal of Clinical Nutrition*, 48, 1988, pp. 152–8.
2. Parthasarathy, S. *et al.*, 'Low-density lipoprotein rich in oleic acid is protected against oxidative modification: implications for dietary prevention of atherosclerosis', *Proceedings of the National Academy of Science*, 87, May 1990, pp. 3894–8.
3. Steinberg, D. *et al.*, 'Beyond cholesterol, modifications of low density lipoprotein that increase its atherogenicity', *New England Journal of Medicine*, 320, 14, pp. 915–23.

Chapter 10

How Much Beta-Carotene Should We Eat?

Beta-carotene has never been given a recommended daily amount (RDA) by either the UK or US governments, and so is not classified as a vitamin. This is because it is not considered to be *essential* to health – without it we do not suffer from deficiency diseases. Without adequate supplies of vitamins we *do* suffer deficiency diseases. Despite being an important source of vitamin A for many people, beta-carotene remains a nutrient which is 'optional' in the eyes of the authorities.

However, statistical evidence that a high intake of dietary fruit and vegetables lowers cancer rates is so strong that major cancer institutions are advising people to eat more fruit and vegetables, especially those rich in beta-carotene. In a recent summing up of the work on beta-carotene to date, Dr R. Ziegler of the American National Cancer Institute writes: '... low intake of vegetables and fruits and carotenoids is consistently associated with an increased risk of lung cancer in both prospective and retrospective studies. In addition, low levels of serum or plasma beta-carotene are consistently associated with the subsequent development of lung cancer. The simplest explanation is that beta-carotene is indeed protective.'[1]

In the same paper Dr Ziegler qualifies this statement by writing: '... the importance of other carotenoids, other constituents of vegetables and fruits, and other nutrients whose levels in the blood are partially correlated with those of beta-carotene has not been adequately explored.' No scientist is prepared to say any more until further comprehensive evidence has been gathered. This long-awaited evidence will come mainly from the intervention trials being funded by the American National Cancer Institute, which is currently carrying out a series of seven trials involving beta-carotene.

Recommendations by Cancer Institutions

Scientists need more concrete proof to establish that beta-carotene does have a role to play in protection against certain cancers. But the fact remains that a high intake of fruits and vegetables is strongly associated with a lower risk of cancer. The mechanism by which this works remains to be established and could be due in part to other common components such as vitamin C. Cancer institutes around the world are recommending that we increase our intake of fresh fruit and vegetables, particularly those that contain beta-carotene. Here is what they say:

1. *The American National Cancer Institute*: 'Scientists who study the foods people in different countries eat are finding that diets rich in beta-carotene and vitamin C are associated with reduced risk for certain cancers. Some research links diets high in vitamin C with reduced risk of cancers of the stomach and oesophagus, and diets low in beta-carotene with increased risk of cancers of the lung, bladder and larynx.'

2. *American Cancer Society*: 'Choose dark green and deep yellow fresh vegetables and fruits as sources of vitamin A, such as carrots, spinach, sweet potatoes, peaches, apricots; and oranges, grapefruit, strawberries, green and red peppers for vitamin C. These foods may help lower risk for cancers of the larynx, oesophagus and the lung.'

3. *Canadian Cancer Society*: 'Canada's Food Guide suggests that you have four to five servings of fruits and vegetables daily. And because vegetables, particularly the leafy green and yellow ones, have more vitamin A, folic acid and iron than fruits, the Food Guide recommends at least two of the servings be vegetables. ... Most of the research to date has related carotene-containing foods with cancer prevention.'

4. *Europe Against Cancer*: 'Frequently eat fresh fruits and vegetables and cereals with high fibre content. There is some evidence that foods rich in pro-vitamin A [i.e. beta-carotene] and vitamin C may give protection against cancer.'

5. *German Society for Nutrition*: 'Cancer risk can probably be reduced by a sufficient intake of vitamin A or its precursor carotene.'

6. *Costa Rica Social Security Nutritional Department*: 'Consume vitamin A and carotenoids.'

A Recommended Daily Amount

A result of so much promising research is that questions begin to be asked about how much beta-carotene should be consumed on a daily basis. The RDA panels in the UK and the US are currently not prepared to award beta-carotene with strict 'vitamin' status, but do not dismiss its potential value. Over the next few years, the British panel will be reviewing the evidence in favour of beta-carotene. It takes the view that if the nutrient could be seen to have a quantifiable health effect then there is no reason why it should not have a status similar to a vitamin. It may not be called a vitamin, but may be part of a second tier of nutrients vital for good health – with more specific dosage recommendations than dietary guidelines.

Professor John Weisburger, Director Emeritus of the American Health Foundation, is prepared to go one step further and suggest that certain groups of the population could benefit from supplementing their diet with beta-carotene and other essential micronutrients. These groups are pregnant women, older people who may have difficulty chewing vegetables and fruits, and those on weight reduction programmes. Out of the general population these people are more likely to have a less healthy nutritional status. As Chapter 3 reported, smokers are also more likely to have lower beta-carotene levels and may benefit from taking a supplement. Don't forget that beta-carotene is a valuable source of vitamin A.

In 1988, a study by American researcher Paul Lachance

looked at how much beta-carotene should be in the diet.[2] His main point of reference was the analysis done by the United States Department of Agriculture (USDA) on its own dietary menus, and on those published by the American National Cancer Institute. USDA calculated the amount of vitamin A activity in an ideal healthy menu and found that it was equal to between 5.2 and 6 mg of beta-carotene daily. From this Lachance concluded: 'If one were following these diets, one would be taking in 5.2 to 6 mg per day of beta-carotene, a range I believe we can justifiably use as a guideline for intake.'

He goes on to say: '... if we follow the USDA or the ANCI guidelines, 90 per cent of our vitamin A intake should be in the form of carotenoids ... 1.5 mg is the level of carotene equivalency currently consumed.' Lachance suggests that Americans should increase their current intakes of beta-carotene fourfold.

15 mg a Day?

Another paper, written by British Professor Anthony Diplock, focuses on the topic of whether the RDA should be increased for certain nutrients, notably the antioxidants vitamin E, vitamin C, beta-carotene and selenium.[3] These nutrients in particular, because they are all antioxidants and could have an important influence over the development of disease states. In his paper, Professor Diplock suggests that low intakes could lead to a higher incidence of disease in which free radicals are involved, such as ischaemic heart disease and other degenerative conditions.

In his conclusion, Professor Diplock suggests that the intake of vitamin C, vitamin E and beta-carotene should be increased. With particular reference to beta-carotene, Professor Diplock links it with the evidence found in favour of its protective effect against lung cancer. He writes: 'cogent reasons are emerging for the recognition of beta-carotene as a vitamin in its own right, independent of its pro-vitamin A role. If this is accepted then an RDA of about 15 mg might be found to be legitimate.'

The figure of 15 mg has not been conjured out of the air; several other papers have used it as a point of reference. Dr J.

Constantino and team researched blood levels of beta-carotene over several years.[4] The results from one year of the study were published in 1988. The paper considered the results from 300 male participants. All of the men were smokers who had smoked 20 cigarettes a day for at least 20 years. 150 men received a placebo, the other 150 received 15 mg daily of beta-carotene.

They found that blood levels of beta-carotene in the latter group rose substantially after two months of supplementation. They continued to rise with several months of treatment reaching a plateau after four months. The findings showed that all participants had substantial increases in beta-carotene as long as they complied with taking the beta-carotene capsules.

The size of the person did make a difference – smaller people had greater increases in blood levels. These levels were also higher for people who had greater concentrations of high-density lipoproteins (HDL) in their blood. More HDL means better protection against furring-up of the arteries (see Chapter 9). None of the men developed carotenodermia (yellowing of the skin) which can be a side-effect of taking beta-carotene longterm.

The study's primary purpose was to find whether a dosage of 15 mg of beta-carotene could be given while avoiding the visual side-effect of carotenodermia. Dr Constantino concludes: 'These findings indicate that if effective against cancer, beta-carotene would be an ideal chemopreventive agent. It is relatively inexpensive, easy to administer, and at least under the conditions of this study has no side-effects.'

The Basel study examined the links between antioxidant vitamins and rates of ischaemic heart disease and cancer.[5] The 1987 paper, written up by Dr Fred Gey, suggested that the dietary supply of essential antioxidants such as vitamins C, E and beta-carotene could vary a person's defence potential against certain diseases. The study showed that low levels of beta-carotene and vitamin A increase the risk of stomach cancer, but if low levels of both nutrients occur simultaneously the risk is even greater; and that low levels of beta-carotene and vitamin E increase the risk of lung cancer.

The paper concludes: '... the presently available data suggest that in order to achieve the potentially maximum prophylactic effect of the essential antioxidants against important health hazards a minimum daily intake can be recommended for beta-carotene of 15 mg, vitamin C of 100 mg, and vitamin E of 60 IU. Even higher intakes may be necessary for optimum health. . . .'

Dosages of beta-carotene used by the American Cancer Institute add weight to the suggestion for an intake of 15 mg or over. The lowest daily dosage used in the NCI's intervention trials is 15 mg daily; the maximum daily dosage is 50 mg. Scientists involved in a major intervention trial looking at beta-carotene have not reported any yellowing of the skin from a dosage of 50 mg every two days.

As mentioned earlier, research that has been done centres around the 15 mg daily level. So, if a person chose to take a supplement, or indeed to eat the equivalent amount of fruit and vegetables (see Chapter 3) this is an amount to aim for in the absence of an official RDA. Collective bodies and individuals are remaining cautious over the 'cancer connection' and level of intake, while advising people to increase their overall intake of beta-carotene-containing foods. Taking a dietary supplement is simply the easy way to maintain levels.

Notes

1. Ziegler, R.G., 'A review of epidemiologic evidence that carotenoids reduce the risk of cancer'. 1989, *Journal of Nutrition*, 119, 1, pp. 116–22.
2. Lachance, P., 'Dietary intake of carotenes and the carotene gap'. *Clinical Nutrition*, 1988, 7, 3, pp. 118–22.
3. Diplock, A.T., 'Dietary supplementation with antioxidants. Is there a case for exceeding the RDA?' *Free Radical Biology and Medicine*, 1987, 39, 3, pp. 199–201.
4. Constantino, J.P., *et. al.*, 'Serum level changes after administration of a pharmacologic dose of beta-carotene'. *American Journal of Clinical Nutrition*, 1988, 48, pp. 1277–83.
5. Gey, F.K., *et. al.*, 'Plasma levels of antioxidant vitamins in relation to ischaemic heart disease and cancer'. *American Journal of Clinical Nutrition*, 1987, 45, pp. 1368–77.

Chapter 11

Ongoing Research into Beta-Carotene

Chemoprevention – the prevention of cancer using natural and synthetic substances in the diet – has spawned worldwide interest; we could have a simple form of medicine which stops cancer in its tracks. As is frequently reported, there are many nutrients which come into this band of classification: vitamins, minerals and types of food. The emphasis is not just on beta-carotene, but on vitamin C, vitamin E, selenium, fat and fibre – a whole range of things we can obtain from our everyday diet.

Research Pointers

Correlations between types of cancer and these factors are first noticed in epidemiological studies. These compile evidence from retrospective trials and dietary observations; for example, how much beta-carotene-rich food does a person eat? When that person is compared to many others do they have a higher or lower risk of developing cancer? This, basically, is how results are arrived at.

These early studies are vital for encouraging further work. Without such a weight of positive evidence, no sponsor would ever be prepared to put up the huge sums of money needed to run more searching trials. There are many animal studies on various nutrients, including beta-carotene, which are also taken into account.

The ethics surrounding animal testing for medical research are extremely controversial, and a high proportion of the public, including some doctors, feel unhappy with the reasoning behind the practice. Nevertheless, many animal models – usually rats, mice and hamsters – have been used to test out theories.

Anti-vivisectionists argue that animals are not as complex as humans and therefore cannot be useful in curing human diseases. Scientists involved in the testing disagree and believe that much can be deduced from these experiments, and the results used as a pointer towards future work in humans. The issue is a thorny one, but as science advances, more humane methods of experimentation are being introduced, such as cell culture testing.

In the case of beta-carotene, both epidemiological and animal studies have pointed towards a possible protective effect of beta-carotene in certain types of cancer, such as lung, mouth and stomach. Animal studies have also seen positive effects in skin, bladder and colon cancer.

Intervention Trials

Intervention trials on beta-carotene and other nutrients are part of the US National Cancer Institute's extensive chemoprevention programme, begun in 1980. In an information paper entitled *Cancer Prevention Research: Chemoprevention and Diet*, the NCI states:

> The goals of chemoprevention research include finding ways to halt or reverse the development of cancer in people already exposed to cancer-causing agents (carcinogens) or potential carcinogens. This strategy may help those people at high risk for cancer as well as those with certain precancerous conditions that might increase their risk of developing cancer.

It goes on to reaffirm its huge practical commitment by saying:

> Information on cancer inhibition comes from studies in tissue culture, animals, and human populations. These studies have identified two groups of potential chemo-preventive agents: naturally occuring substances found in

many foods, and synthetic compounds considered safe for clinical trials. These include naturally occurring forms of vitamin A, the retinoids – synthetic derivatives and chemical 'cousins' of vitamin A – and vitamin A's precursors, beta-carotene and other carotenoids. Vitamin A and beta-carotene, and other carotenoids . . . Other chemopreventive agents include vitamin C . . . vitamin E . . . vitamin B_{12} and the B vitamin folate . . . and the trace metal selenium.

A further reason for research is that 40 per cent of American adults now take vitamin supplements. By implication, through running intervention trials, the NCI will be able to determine benefits of supplements, and possible harm from excessive use.

In 1981, the NCI established the first human intervention trials. In the words of W.D. De Wys and colleagues:

Clinical trials are utilized to clarify the specificity of epidemiological studies to determine which animal model results are applicable to humans, to evaluate toxicity and risk benefit relationships and to determine the feasibility of applying a given preventive intervention to the population at large.[1]

The NCI is currently supporting seven intervention trials looking specifically at beta-carotene. Three of them have over 20,000 participants, and are viewed as the trials that will make or break beta-carotene. They are not just based in America but stretch to Finland and China (see Figure 11.1).

All these studies are carried out over a number of years and have been carefully structured beforehand through preliminary trials. Each study will have a group of groups taking the chemopreventive agent(s) and another group given a placebo (a capsule that looks the same but doesn't actually do anything). All groups will be carefully monitored to make sure that they are actually taking their treatments.

You will notice that some of these studies – such as the one in China – use a combination of nutrients. This is because researchers wish to see whether beta-carotene can work in

Site of study	Agent	Study population
Lung	Vitamin E Beta-carotene	Cigarette smokers
Lung	Beta-carotene Retinoids	Cigarette smokers
Colon	Beta-carotene	Those with previous colon tumour
All sites	Beta-carotene	Healthy doctors
Skin	Beta-carotene	Tanzanian albinos
Lung	Retinol	Men exposed to asbestos
Oesophagus	Multivitamins Vitamin A Vitamin C Vitamin E Zinc Selenium Molybdenum Niacin Riboflavin Beta-carotene	Chinese people

Source: National Cancer Institute, USA

Figure 11.1: Beta-carotene intervention trials currently running.

harmony with other substances, such as vitamin E. Many experts in the beta-carotene field refuse to dismiss the synergistic role played by other nutrients.

This is a very sensible approach, as the links between beta-carotene and cancers have been seen in the diet, and the diet consists of far more than beta-carotene. Even fruits and vegetables rich in beta-carotene contain other non-nutrients such as flavones (plant pigments) and indoles (chemicals used for plant growth).

While the studies are taking place, researchers must keep a watchful eye over participants to ensure that they follow the regime of treatment. Regular tests of nutrient levels in the bloodstream are an essential part of this practice. In recent years the technology which can be used to measure carotenoids in the bloodstream has improved dramatically, with the introduction of high performance liquid chromatography (HPLC). The tests show in detail the levels of carotenoids circulating in the blood, indicating whether a participant has been taking his/her dosage regularly. Of course, in the trials looking at the effects of beta-carotene, levels in the blood should be elevated in the groups being supplemented.

Further Advances in Intervention

In most of the beta-carotene trials mentioned, the endpoint is the development of full-blown cancer. When the trial has finished the number of cancer occurrences are compared in the groups being given the active agent and the groups on a placebo. However, the latest cancer research suggests that 'cancer risk is associated with detectable changes in genetic structure'.[2]

Micronuclei (formed when a cell's nucleus splinters) have been observed to be an early indicator of genetic change – itself indicative of a pre-cancerous state. Studies conducted by Professor Hans Stich (see Chapter 7) show that micronuclei occur in mouth cancer, found widely in South America and Asia as a result of the chewing of betel nut leaves. A reduction in the amount of micronuclei in mouth cells can be stimulated by supplementation with beta-carotene and vitamin A.

The Big Three – Specific Intervention Trials

The NCI is involved with three very influential studies: the Hennekens Trial, the Lin Xian Trial and the ATBC Trial.

Participants number over 80,000 in total – a colossal group of people to be involved in the research of such a relatively narrow field. It is hoped that when the last of the three – the Hennekens Trial in 1995 – finishes results will show either a clear positive or negative response in relation to beta-carotene and cancer prevention. Let us look at the trials in more detail.

1. The Hennekens Trial

Based in the United States, the trial has 22,071 male participants and will run until 1995. It is named after Harvard medical School's Professor Charles Hennekens, who is in charge of the study. The trial is looking for links between beta-carotene intake and cancers at all sites.

Dr Richard Peto, one of Britain's top epidemiologists, who first suggested that beta-carotene could be used in chemo-prevention in 1981, considers this study to be excellent.[3] Meticulously designed to take into account all variables, the trial will give either a positive result in favour of beta-carotene, or an 'informed no'.

The trial began in 1982, initially to look into the proposition that aspirin could stop heart disease. As the participants, male doctors between the ages of 40 and 84, could only be given an aspirin every other day for safety factors, it was decided to include another substance for research.

The study directors chose beta-carotene, due to the scientific excitement caused by the 1981 paper produced by Peto and colleagues. The aspirin part of the study has now been concluded, but the beta-carotene part is being continued until 1995. It has already been extended once because of lack of cancer development.

This study is interesting because the doctors were all fit and healthy at the beginning and were not classified as a 'high-risk' cancer group. Women were not invited to join the trial; first because at the time only one out of ten US doctors was female; and second because their rate of heart disease is only a third that suffered by men, and the reduction of heart disease was the primary hypothesis in the trial.

Every other day, the doctors must take 50 mg of synthetic beta-carotene. While the branches of the study were running simultaneously the doctors were split into four groups. The first took buffered aspirin and beta-carotene; the second took buffered aspirin and beta-carotene placebo; the third group took aspirin placebo and beta-carotene; while the fourth and last group took placebos of both. As mentioned in the previous chapter, the consumption of beta-carotene has already resulted in a 50 per cent reduction in heart disease, compared with the control group; a tremendous and unexpected boost for beta-carotene. The results of the cancer trial are yet to come.

No skin yellowing caused by the regular intake of beta-carotene has been observed in any of the doctors. Participants are monitored by counting the number of tablets taken, and by regular blood tests, to find out the circulating levels of beta-carotene. From blood samples taken at the beginning of the trial the researchers will be able to see who was low on beta-carotene to begin with. The results of this study will be of major significance in the field of chemoprevention.

2. The Lin Xian Trial

This study is based in the county of Lin Xian, in the province of Heinan, north China. It has the highest number of participants out of the three big trials – 33,400 men and women. Organized by the Institute of Chinese Medical Sciences, and co-ordinated by Dr Bill Blott of the NCI, the study is looking at beta-carotene and other nutrients in relation to risk of cancer of the oesophagus.

In Lin Xian the rate of oesophageal cancer is one of the highest in the world – one in three inhabitants will develop it. A number of possible causes have been suggested: fermented foods, pickled vegetables, and cigarette smoking. In general these people have a very low intake of foods rich in beta-carotene, vitamin C and the B vitamins. The aim of the trial is to bring the participants' nutrient status up to the top 10 per cent of the US population, among the most well-fed people in the world.

The trial has been running since 1985, and the participants are half women and half men, aged between 40 and 69. There are two branches of the Lin Zian Trial. The first involves 3,400 people, and aims to see whether daily supplementation with 25 different vitamins and minerals will reduce the occurrence of oesophageal dysplasia – the pre-cancerous state. For the group being supplemented, their daily dose includes vitamin A, vitamin C, zinc, selenium, magnesium, and 15 mg of beta-carotene.

The second trial involves the remaining resource of 30,000 people, divided into eight different groups which between them are taking various combinations of vitamin A and zinc, niacin and riboflavin, vitamin C and molybdenum, selenium and vitamin E, and beta-carotene. One group gets all four combinations, six groups get two, and the last group is given placebos.

In total, 15,000 people will be taking beta-carotene every day. Supplements are distributed each month and consumption checked. Blood specimens are taken every three months to ensure that participants are complying. The trial is due to end in 1991 and will not give such clear-cut results as the Hennekens Trial because its scope of chemopreventive agents is much wider. However, if a strong nutritional status proves to stave off cancer of the oesophagus, the research will be hailed as a breakthrough, because the sample size is so large, and it is relevant to women as well as men.

3. The ATBC (Alpha Tocopherol/ Beta-Carotene) Study

Based in Finland and organized by the National Public Health Institute in Helsinki, the trial is overseen by Professor Heinonen. Participants number 29,246 male smokers, who are being supplemented beta-carotene and vitamin E. The trial is seeking to find an association between these nutrients and lung cancer.

The ATBC Trial has been running since 1985, the men chosen to take part are aged between 50 and 69. It was decided to concentrate on men because, at the time, so few Finnish women smoked. (Although the rates for female smoking are now rising steadily.)

The researchers chose vitamin E as the second chemo-preventive agent because, at the time, the data available put it in a more favourable light than vitamin C or selenium. It also makes economic sense to study two substances in one trial because of the sheer expense of organization.

The participants have been divided into four groups; one is taking 20 mg of beta-carotene daily, one is taking 50 mg of vitamin E daily, one group is taking both daily, and the last group is being given a placebo. The trial is due to finish in the spring of 1993 and results should be available by 1994. The outcome is of prime interest to cancer researchers because the supplementation is being given to people in a high risk group – possibly making the suggested protective role of the beta-carotene even more difficult. If the results prove positive the trial would have a dramatic effect on the treatment of lung cancer; beta-carotene could be prescribed as a medicine to those in high risk groups.

Some Bad Results

The three trials discussed above are very exciting, and could be hailed as a momentous breakthrough in the prevention of cancer if results are positive. But two intervention trials using beta-carotene have demonstrated very disappointing results.

As was recently reported in the *Journal of the National Cancer Institute*, a nine-month trial designed to observe the effect of beta-carotene and retinoic acid (a vitamin A derivative) on oral leukoplakia (pre-cancerous state in mouth) showed that the retinoic acid worked but the beta-carotene did not. Despite the poor results, Dr Lippman commented: 'It is not a question of "now beta-carotene is dead" . . . In this specific study designed to answer this specific question, it didn't work.'[4]

In the same article, another study overseen by Dr Robert Greenberg of the Norris Cotton Cancer Centre in New Hampshire, is reported to have shown negative results when using a daily dose of 50 mg beta-carotene to try to prevent the recurrence of skin cancer. Dr Greenberg also feels that this bad result does not signify the end of the road for beta-carotene, and that it is too early to dismiss it as ineffective.

Worth Waiting For?

The world of science can be a frustrating one. Progress can be slow and contradictory. The temptation is to jump to conclusions and simplify results. When a scientist has spent forty years looking into the hopeful possibilities of one nutrient, failures can be very hard to comprehend. But in the words of Professor Krinsky of Tufts University, Boston, who has done just that with beta-carotene, that is the nature of science. This decade could herald an enormous breakthrough in the fight against cancer, using simple, painless techniques, or it could herald a huge disappointment. In general, the carotenoid story is far from over: investigation into beta-carotene has led to research into lutein, lycopene and alpha-carotene. As the heart disease part of the Hennekens Trial shows, you can never predict what science will discover. Whether or not the cancer hunch proves true, one thing is assured. The status of beta-carotene as a safe and useful nutrient is assured.

Notes

1. De Wys, W.D. *et al.*, 'Clinical trials in cancer prevention', *Cancer*, 58, 1986, pp. 1954–62.
2. Malone, W.F., 'Studies evaluating antioxidants and beta-carotene as chemopreventives', The NCI, Chemoprevention Branch.
3. Peto, R. *et al.*, 'Can dietary beta-carotene materially reduce human cancer rates?', *Nature*, 290, 1981, pp. 201–8.
4. Smigel, K., 'Beta-carotene didn't prevent cancer: what's up, Doc?', *Journal of the National Cancer Institute*, 82, 11, 1990, pp. 899–900.

Index